W9-CGU-899

# The New York Book of Beauty

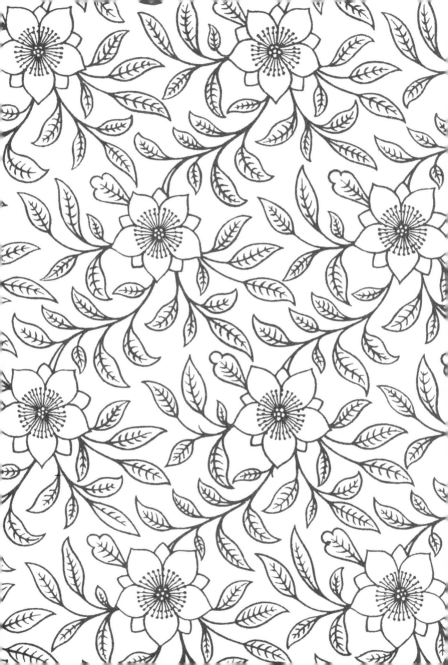

# The
# New York
# Book
# of
# Beauty

&

Deborah
Blumenthal

CITY & COMPANY

NEW YORK

To Annie, Sophie, and Ralph

Copyright © 1995 by Deborah Blumenthal
Cover illustration copyright © 1995 by Gladys Perint Palmer

All rights reserved. No portion of this book may be reproduced
without written permission from the publisher.

City & Company
22 West 23rd Street
New York, NY 10010

Printed in the United States of America

Design by Leah Lococo

Library of Congress Cataloging-in-Publication Data is available upon request.

ISBN 1-885492-23-5
First Edition

PUBLISHER'S NOTE: Neither City & Company nor the author has
any interest, financial or personal, in the locations listed in this book. No fees
were paid or services rendered in exchange for inclusion in these pages.

Please also note that every effort was made to ensure that
information regarding addresses, phone numbers, hours, and prices
was accurate and up-to-date at the time of publication.

# Contents

Introduction 6

Beauty Supplies and Fragrances: Where to Get Them 8

Hair 32
Scissor Wizards 33
Color Czars 43
Hair Helpers 52
Adding On: Wigs & Hair Extensions 54
Taking It Off: Electrolysis 57

Saving Face: Skin care & Makeup 60

Manicure Masters 70

Workout Whereabouts 78

Massage Mavens 94

Day Spas 106

Department Store Beauty 112

Beauty on a Budget 122

Introduction

NEW YORK IS A BEAUTY MECCA. It draws a dizzying array of hairdressers, makeup artists, estheticians, manicurists, and massage therapists, who hold court in salons, spas, gyms, and boutiques zigzagging uptown, downtown, and midtown. Help is everywhere to be found. But who are the best, and how do you sift through the possibilities? Where do you shop for beauty products? Whom do you entrust with changing your hair style and hair color, enhancing your makeup, or kneading away your tension?

To find out, I asked the experts *about* the experts.

Almost one hundred top haircutters, colorists, massage therapists, makeup artists, manicurists, beauty writers, modeling-agency directors, and compulsive bargain-hunters shared their secrets. They told me whom they use, whom they respect, and where they shop. Then I followed their leads. I went to the stores and pharmacies, looked at products and tested them, had manicures, pedicures, scalp treatments, massages, and facials, tried cutters and colorists, visited salons, went to classes, and walked through gyms—just the type of legwork I have always done in my 15 years as a beauty and health writer. (The only shopping sources not included are the discount drugstores; these are found throughout the city, and need no introduction.)

THE NEW YORK BOOK OF BEAUTY is a streamlined, road-tested tour through New York City's vast beauty landscape. It represents a wide spectrum of services in Manhattan, the part of the city with the greatest concentration of salons and practitioners. It looks at beauty at all price levels—even where to get makeup and services *gratis*. It's a beauty Baedeker for all, whatever their beauty needs.

DEBORAH BLUMENTHAL

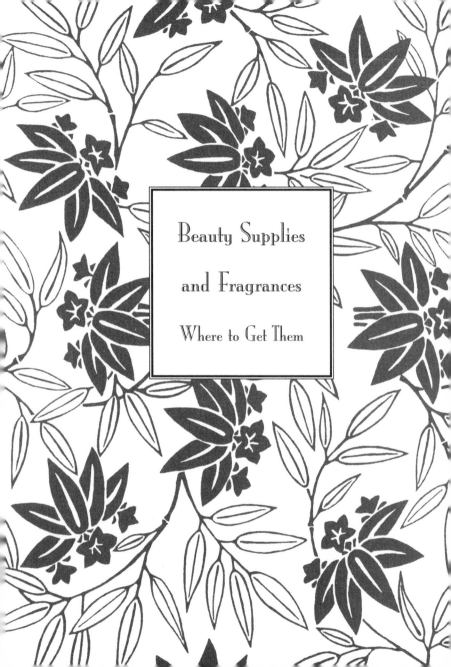

Beauty Supplies

and Fragrances

Where to Get Them

# Alcone

235 W. 19th St. (212) 633-0551

Hours: Monday through Friday 11 AM–6 PM; Saturday 12 PM–5 PM

If you love makeup, this small, unpretentious theatrical makeup supplier is the real McCoy. Makeup artists, models, and actresses shop here, as do those who like to experiment with brands not found in drug and department stores. Alcone regulars know that they don't even have to visit the store—they can get products by mail through the very detailed catalog. You may want to pass on the Paramount Death Green powder formulated for zombies, and the gel wound kits (ugh!), but not the light, fresh-smelling Visiora foundation made by Dior, a favorite of models: 1 oz. bottle, $29.

Other top sellers are the R.C.M.A. creme foundation (good coverage); LeClerc powders, highly opaque and a good base if your skin is clear, $35 for the small size, and cheaper than you'd find uptown; the German Kryolan mini lip palettes with 14 colors for $14.20, or the larger palettes with 12 for $24.70; empty makeup palettes; professional brushes; and roomy makeup boxes.

There are numerous professional brands here: William Tuttle, Joe Blasco, Bob Kelly, Kryolan, Cinema Secret, R.C.M.A., Ben Nye, to name just a few. Have questions about color, consistency, formulation? Behind-the-counter makeup artist Becky Browner is an expert.

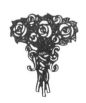

# Aveda Aromatherapy Esthetique

509 Madison Ave., bet. 52nd and 53rd Sts.  (212) 832-2416
Hours: Monday through Friday 10 AM–7 PM;
Saturday 10 AM–6 PM; Sunday 12 PM–5 PM
456 West Broadway, bet. Prince and Houston Sts.  (212) 473-0280
Hours: Monday through Saturday 11 AM–8 PM; Sunday 12 PM–6 PM

Aveda is an environmentally friendly company whose cosmetics are largely plant-derived. In addition to makeup, it sells exotic-sounding "balancing infusions," "purescriptions," and shampoos with yummy ingredients: Madder Root shampoo, for example, contains (in addition to madder root) red clover, aloe, almond, and cherry bark.

Hair products have a particularly strong following. One of the best-selling shampoos is Shampure. You can try a 50 ml bottle for $2.70, or a liter for $20.50. Other shampoos are designed for specific hair colors to emphasize highlights (Shhh! Don't tell: When Giorgio Armani visited the Soho emporium, he bought the Blue Malva shampoo, which brightens gray hair).

The shops also sell scented candles; straw gift boxes perfect for storing makeup, $6; a back brush with soft, rubber massaging fingers on the flip side, $20; and even "Comforting Tea," in a 4 oz. brown glass bottle for $12.

Hair and skin treatments are given upstairs. A 90-minute body massage costs $95, and the popular stress-relieving scalp treatment with essential oils costs $45 for 30 minutes.

# C.O. Bigelow Chemists

414 Ave. of the Americas, bet. 8th and 9th Sts.  (212) 533-2700
MAIL ORDER: 1-800-793-5433
Hours: Monday through Friday 7:30 AM–9 PM
Saturday 8:30 AM–5:30 PM; Sunday 8:30 AM–5:30 PM

If you look back fondly on the days before drugstore megagiants took the place of user-friendly neighborhood pharmacies, head down to this Greenwich Village landmark. Established in 1838, Bigelow prides itself on service and goes far beyond aspirin and bandages. Exotic European cosmetics are its forte, along with homeopathic remedies (it claims to have the city's biggest supply), aromatherapy oils, shaving paraphernalia, makeup bags, hair accessories, and costume jewelry.

Like exotic toothpastes?  Bigelow carries the his-and-her Italian Marvis brand, gorgeously packaged, $7.95; Email Diamant Red Toothpaste which tints the gums red so the teeth look whiter, $6.95; Fluocaril's spaceage-looking toothbrushes, $7.95; LeClerc face powder; Valobra soaps from the 200year-old Genoa factory; Mustela baby products from France for those eager to take a status step up from J&J; and Avigal Hennas. Bigelow delivers throughout Manhattan, and will mail, or send via UPS or Federal Express.

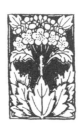

# The Body Shop

14 New York locations, including Queens and Staten Island
For store information, to order products by mail, or request
a catalog: 1-800-541-2535

If you fancy products like Banana Hair Conditioner, Peppermint Foot
Lotion, and Mango Body Butter, and you're an eco-friendly consumer, welcome to Nirvana.

This worldwide mega beauty operation was started in England
in 1976 by earth mother/entrepreneur Anita Roddick. Now the
operation has blossomed to 45 countries and over 1,100 branches.
Roddick's original 25-product line has grown to over 400 products
and more than 500 accessories.

The enticing offerings in fresh, brightly colored packaging
include hair—and skin—care products and cosmetics whose names
will positively whet your appetite: Tangerine Beer Shampoo,
Avocado Body Butter, Watermelon Suncare products, and Brazil
Nut Conditioner, plus toothpaste in cinnamint or fennel.

Some best–sellers: The White Musk fragrance products; Cocoa
Butter Hand and Body Lotion; Vitamin-E Cream; Banana
Conditioner; Peppermint Foot Lotion; and Black Mascara. Makeup
sales are booming, and one of the most versatile products is the all-
in-one stick called Complete Colour, $9.95. This cream dries to a
powder and can be used as eye shadow, blusher, or lipstick.

# Boyd's of Madison Avenue

655 Madison Ave., bet. 60th and 61st Sts. (212) 838-6558
1-800-683-BOYD
Hours: Monday through Friday 8:30 AM–7 PM (makeovers start at 9 AM); Saturday 9:30 AM–6:30 PM; Sunday 12 PM–6 PM

First impression: hair care heaven. Counters spill over with hairbrushes, combs, barrettes, headbands, and accessories. Poke around—you'll find a fabulous collection of makeup mirrors made in France by Arpin, $25 to $900.

Move to the middle of the store and you'll come to the makeup counter, a black granite rectangle bearing makeover ammunition. Sit down on a counter stool, buy four products, and you'll be entitled to a makeover, including a how-to diagram to take home. Makeovers are big business here; there are nine full-time cosmeticians who do a couple of hundred a week. They work with Boyd's own Renoir cosmetics, which are priced on the high side (as is just about everything in the store): matte oil-free makeup, $23.50; eye shadows, Extra Heavy Mascara (Cher's a fan); and lipsticks, all $14.75.

A great mail service: If you have a lipstick you'd like to match, need a new blush, or are trying to find an eye shadow to replace a discontinued one, just send them a color swatch and they'll match it. Or give them a sketch of an accessory you're looking for—anything from an earring to a handbag—and they'll try to find it.

Need your makeup done for a wedding or other special occasion? Home or office visits cost $100.

# Cambridge Chemists

21 E. 65th St. (212) 734-5678

Hours: Monday through Friday 9:30 AM–7 PM; Saturday 10 AM–5 PM

If you're more the old world apothecary-shopper than the Duane Reade bargain-hunter, this elegant, dark-paneled pharmacy is for you. It's home to exotic European soaps, cosmetics, badger shaving brushes, and various cosmeceuticals. And the operative word here is "service."

"If it's sitting on a drugstore shelf in London today, I can have it here by courier tomorrow," says Joseph Policar, the low-key pharmacist/owner. The store networks with pharmacies in Paris, London, St. Martin, and Martinique, and it's often the first to introduce European products.

Cambridge carries the hard-to-find Yardley shaving soaps (in fact, the shop claims to have the country's biggest selection of shaving soaps); natural sponges from Greece; colorfully packaged jumbo 12 oz. Portuguese soaps by Brito, $12.50; an amazing array of badger shaving brushes, $49.50–$500; products by Floris, Trumper, Innoxa, and Cyclax; and LeClerc face powders (the banana shade works for everyone in New York, Mr. LeClerc says).

There are some exotic cosmeceuticals, such as the Vitamin K Formula Clarifying Cream, which promises to improve the appearance of bruises; and Sil-K, silicone sheeting (by prescription) that claims to improve keloid and hypertrophic scars. Policar promises to work with your physician to make any prescription you need. Products can be mailed or messengered.

# Caswell-Massey

518 Lexington Ave. at 48th St. (212) 755-2254
MAIL ORDER: 1-800-326-0500
Hours: Monday through Friday 9 AM–7 PM; Saturday 10 AM–6 PM

Where did George Washington and Buffalo Bill buy their cologne? Who whipped up Sarah Bernhardt's own night cream? Who developed Greta Garbo's personal fragrance? You guessed it.

Caswell-Massey, "America's Oldest Chemists and Perfumers" (dating from 1752), has been making cosmetics and fragrances infused with spices, herbs, and essential oils before it was cosmetically correct to do so. And if you derive comfort from shopping where legendary figures of government and the arts have shopped, go no further.

CM developed and still sells Number Six Cologne, Washington's favorite; "My Own," which was Garbo's fragrance; Casma, the scent used by Gloria Swanson and Carole Lombard; Almond Cold Cream Soap, used by Eisenhower; and Jockey Club Cologne, favored by JFK. The Presidential Soap Collection, containing Number Six, Almond Cold Cream, and Jockey Club, costs $25.

# Cosmair Beauty Response Center

575 Fifth Ave., corner of 47th St., 8th floor (212) 984-4164
Hours: Monday through Friday 9 AM–4 PM, occasional evenings

If you're into being a guinea pig, and are willing to help Cosmair evaluate cosmetics or fragrances (L'Oréal, Lancôme), you'll be thanked with free products. Women in the tri-state area 18 years of age and up can take part in testing panels by calling and making an appointment to fill out a demographic profile.

If you're accepted, you'll take part in a session lasting 30–45 minutes. Those testing products must be willing to come back at least once to report results. After each visit, participants receive a gift of products. If the testing requires three visits, the gift of highest value is given after the third visit.

## Cosmetics Plus
15 Manhattan locations
For information on nearest locations: (212) 319-2120
Hours: Seven days. Call for hours.

This cosmetics giant offers discounts on many major lines of cosmetics and fragrances, ranging from the more usual 10–15 percent to as high as 75 percent on specials. The chain claims to have the largest collection of fragrances and cosmetics in the world (it doesn't carry Estée Lauder), including some hard to find lines, such as Payot. It will meet any published price of a product, and offers special bonuses to those who become members of the store's club. No price quotes over the phone.

# Cosmetic Show

919 Third Ave. at 56th St.  (212) 750-8418
Hours: Monday through Friday 8 AM–7 PM; Saturday 10 AM–5 PM;
Sunday 11 AM–5 PM

This is a place you hear about from bargain-loving friends—you'd never find it on your own. It's easily missed from the street because there are no signs or product-stocked windows. Walk to the entrance of this black-glass office building, but don't go in. Turn left and you'll see double doors. One says "Cosmetics, Fragrances." You've found it.

Cosmetic Show sells products from many prestigious lines at such low prices your jaw will drop. Erno Laszlo Normalizer Shake-it, a foundation that retails for $30, is $9 here. A $12 bar of Laszlo Hydra Therapy soap sells for $2.50. Lancome lip pencils (if you're lucky enough to find a shade you like) sell for $4, and there's a very limited number of Lancôme polishes for $5. Revlon polish costs $2, so do L'Oréal lipsticks. Elizabeth Arden's Millennium Throat Renewal Creme, regularly $49, costs $24.

Also here: a great selection of makeup bags for $5, and tote bags for about $10. The stock includes fragrances for men and women, and gift items such as a pewter-toned Polo shaving mug by Ralph Lauren that is marked $60—but sells here for $8.

Of course, you have to be lucky. Color selection is often limited, and so is the number of items from any one company. Those who get the best bargains come  often and check for what's just off the truck. Another plus: Prices include tax!

# Crabtree & Evelyn

620 Fifth Ave. at Rockefeller Center  (212) 581-5022
520 Madison Ave. at 53rd St.  (212) 758-6419
151 World Trade Center, concourse level  (212) 432-7134
1310 Madison Avenue, corner of 93rd St. (212) 289-3923
Hours: Monday through Saturday 10 AM–6 PM

If you stay at four-star hotels when you travel, you're probably familiar with the fruit- and flower-infused products made by Crabtree & Evelyn. But you don't have to leave home to find them. These four Manhattan shops sell the popular creams, lotions, soaps, bath products, candles, and potpourri in Victorian design packaging and scented with the essences of rose, violet, freesia, gardenia, lavender, lemon, lime, lily of the valley, carnation, almond oil, apricot, aloe vera, apple, and chamomile. Prices are moderate—usually no more than $17—and the bottles look great on bathroom shelves. Two of the most appealing products are the vanilla body lotion, $13, and the almond oil body lotion, $11.50.

# Face Stockholm

224 Columbus Ave. at 71st St.  (212) 769-1420
Hours: Monday through Saturday 11 AM–7 PM; Sunday 12 PM–6 PM

Face Stockholm is the Estée Lauder of Sweden, and has been sold there for 15 years. The makeup is top-notch, and the prices down-to-earth. Model Naomi Campbell's a regular here, and so are a host of other models, actresses, and hip West Siders.

Standouts: The oil-free matte foundation, $16; the mint-toned concealer that banishes redness, $9; the yellow-based concealer stick that hides dark under-eye circles, $7; and pigment-rich eye shadows, $12. Some best-sellers here are the eggplant mascara and cake eyeliner. These shades work for everybody, so buy them if they're in stock—they're usually not.

The store also sells a skin-treatment line, does makeovers, and offers consultations. You can even get an over-the-phone consultation (works for most products, except foundation) and have the products mailed to you. The shop can arrange for freelance makeup artists to do bridal parties.

## 5th Avenue Perfumes, Inc.
M&D DISTRIBUTORS, INC.
246 Fifth Ave. at 28th St. (212) 213-9321
Hours: Seven days 9 AM–7 PM

This tightly packed fragrance shop offers rock-bottom prices on top fragrances. Expect discounts in the 50–70 percent range: a 3.4 oz. Fendi eau de toilette that retails in department stores for $50 costs $22 here; a 1.7 oz. Opium by Yves St. Laurent, which retails at $52, costs $26. Just don't expect service; but at these prices—who cares? No price quotes over the phone.

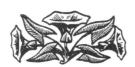

# Laura Geller Makeup Studios

1044 Lexington Ave. at 74th St. (212) 570-5477
Hours: Monday, Tuesday, Wednesday, Friday 10 AM-6:30 PM;
Thursday 10 AM–8 PM; Saturday 10 AM–6:30 PM

Hurrah for the soft, flattering lights, pink walls, pink and tan marble floor, fuscia curtains. This doesn't look like New York. Then out comes Geller, and she's F-R-I-E-N-D-L-Y. Is this Atlanta? Houston? No, this definitely is New York, Geller's town, where she started out doing the makeup of Broadway stars. Her studio is a home-of-sorts to all, whether they're in the shop just to pick up a lipstick or spend a full day having the works: haircut, color, a facial, electrolysis, a makeup lesson, an hour-long individual eyelash application (yes, some people still do that), or even a dress rehearsal makeup application before a big occasion. Geller does a lot of wedding parties, but these services don't come cheap.

Bridal makeup application at the bride's preferred location costs $200. Hair is another $200. Each additional person in the bridal party having their hair done costs $90. Other services and products are more reasonable. Hour-long makeup lessons are $50—with Geller, $75; deep-cleansing facial, $60; 15-minute electrolysis, $20, one hour, $70. The salon also offers advanced glycolic-acid facials done by RN Joan Dalall, the nurse Jackie Onassis used after her plastic surgery.

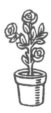

# H2O Plus

650 Madison Ave at 60th St. (212) 750-8119
World Financial Center, 200 Vesey St. (212) 571-6338
805 Third Ave. at 50th St. (212) 832-7020
Hours: Seven days. Call for hours.

These are fun stores to visit, with their bubbling water displays, colorful bottles of cosmetics, and accessories, such as neon–pink loofah gloves. The products come with minimal packaging, are not animal–tested, and are water–rather than oil-based. The line contains over 400 products for women, men, and children, and prices are moderate. Cosmetics range from $5 to $12; bath and shower products from $9.50 to $12.50; and body and aromatherapy items from $6.75 to $38.

# Kiehl's

109 Third Ave., bet. 13th and 14th Sts. (212) 677-3171/(212) 475-3698
1-800-KIEHLS-1 or 1-800-KIEHLS-2
Hours: Monday to Friday 10 AM–6 PM; Saturday 10 AM–4:30 PM

This downtown old world pharmacy with dusty, unkempt windows has a solid uptown following. The hand-blended, herbal-based products in generic plastic bottles also have an old world appeal, but with today's prices. The shop is a kick to visit, even if you could care less about cosmetics. Planes and motorcycles were the favorite toys of the late Aaron Morse, a World War II fighter pilot who owned the shop with his daughter Jami—now CEO—and her husband Klaus

Heidegger. Morse's collection of Harley-Davidsons are on display in an area adjacent to the store that is a kind of kooky museum of family hobbies.

Kiehl's line of products dates back to 1851 (the Morse family bought the shop in 1921) and includes skin-care products, shaving creams, shampoos, conditioners, talc, suntan cream, makeup, perfume essences, cologne, and, most recently, baby products. (Do you believe $33.50 for a 4 oz. diaper-area ointment?) Sales people "advise" instead of "sell," and they're happy to give you samples before you buy.

While Kiehl's no longer offers such nostrums of the past as "Success Oil" or "Money-Drawing Oil," some of the current favorites are the Ultra Facial Moisturizer, $11.50 for 2 ozs.; Creme with Silk Groom for hair, $15.50 for 4 ozs.; Placenta Hair Conditioner and Grooming Aid, $15.95 for 8 ozs.; and Imperiale Repairateur Moisturizing Masque, $19.50 for 1 oz.

## Kris Cosmetics & Fragrances, Inc.
1170 Broadway at 28th St. (212) 213-5788
Hours: Seven days 9:30 AM–8 PM

The service is cut-and-dried here, but prices on designer fragrances are about half of what you'd pay retail. If your favorite fragrance is on the shelf, stock up.

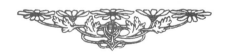

# M.A.C. on Christopher

14 Christopher St. (212) 243-4150

MAIL ORDER: 1-800-387-6707

Hours: Monday through Saturday 12 PM–7 PM; Sunday 1 PM–6 PM

Blaring music assaults your ears in this West Village makeup store. Attempts to reach the makeup displays are futile—customers are three-deep at the counter. None of the black-leather-clad makeup artists are free; they're all painting faces.

Is it worth the wait? Is the makeup so special? No, but it *is* good, definitely good. Plus it's pigment-rich, long-lasting, and comes in a vast range of colors. The Princess of Wales is a fan, as are Madonna (Russian Red lipstick was created for her), Mariah Carey, models Linda Evangelista and Yasmin Le Bon, Michelle Pfeiffer, Liza Minnelli, Roseanne, and on and on.

M.A.C. (Makeup Art Cosmetics) is the brainchild of Frank Toskan, a former hairdresser and photographer who started the company in Toronto in 1984, originally as an outlet for a professional line. Today it's a multimillion-dollar gold mine with plans to expand overseas.

What's everyone buying? Spice lip pencil (the store sells between 700 and 1,000 a month); Mocha lipstick; Twig, a natural brown; Diva, a deep brownish wine; and the deep brown-red Viva Glam. Proceeds from the latter go to helping those with AIDS.

Prices: $12 for lipsticks; $10 for eye shadows; $17.50 for matte foundation. M.A.C. also makes a line of professional foundations called Studio Line which gives full coverage, contains sunscreen, and is waterproof.

# The Make-Up Center

150 W. 55th St. (212) 977-9494

Hours: Monday, Tuesday, Wednesday, Friday 10 AM–6 PM;
Thursday 10 AM–8 PM; Saturday 10 AM–5 PM

The theatrical crowd considers this the best place in midtown to find a wide range of stage makeup (Mehron, Stein's, Bob Kelly, and Ben Nye). Tourists and other ordinary mortals know this long-established makeup shop as a place to find top-quality cosmetics at reasonable prices. The Make-Up Center sells its own product line, and among the best-sellers are the water-based liquid foundation, $14.75; "Fifth Avenue" red lipstick, $9.75; "Gramercy Park," a light orange-brown lipstick, $9.75; and Derma Cover, a thick concealing cream that plastic surgeons recommend to cover bruising, $17.50. Also offered: makeup lessons, manicures, pedicures, facials, and makeup for bridal parties.

# Origins

402 West Broadway, corner of Spring St. (212) 219-9764

Hours: Seven days 11 AM–7 PM

The Origins concept is basically save the earth married to "look and feel your best," and toward that end this Lauder-owned Soho boutique invites touching, testing, smelling, and having fun with cosmetics, bath accessories, unusual soaps, honeys, massage aids, olive oils, aromatherapy products, and a cornucopia of other novel items.

The place has a fresh, clean look, with environmentally friendly white maple, Shaker-style display units, green slate floor tiles, and low-voltage lighting. On display are skin-treatment products, including the skin-care line based on five "skin care pairs"—different pairs for different skin types. The adjacent freestanding cosmetics island holds cosmetics samples, making testing tempting. The cosmetics and sensory-therapy products (not animal-tested or derived) cost $8.50–$25.

One unique twist: foundations come in three formulas, Sheer, More, and Most, depending on coverage needs. You can buy the same color in all three and be prepared for changes in weather and skin condition.

If you're a believer in the powers of plant oils, you'll be enchanted to find products such as Jump Start, a body wash made with "nature's spark plugs," including Ceylon cinnamon, Chinese geranium oil, lavender, and ylang ylang (to "charge your batteries"); Midnight Oil, an eye-opening "inhalations oil" for those who burn the candle at both ends; and a favorite of Origins devotees, Peace of Mind, a peppermint-infused lotion that is dotted on areas around the face to melt away tension.

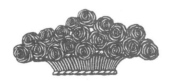

# Perfumania

Seven Manhattan locations:

755 Broadway, corner of 8th St. (212) 979-7674

2321 Broadway, corner of 84th St. (212) 595-8778

782 Lexington Ave., bet. 60th and 61st Sts. (212) 750-2810

342 Madison, corner of 43rd St. (212) 338-0146

1 Penn Plaza, 34th St. at 8th Ave. (212) 268-0049

1 Times Square (212) 944-2311

20 W. 34th St. (212) 736-0414

Hours: Call for individual store hours.

This nationwide chain of 170 stores boasts a stock of 350 fragrances, ranging from the latest top designer scents to hard-to-find oldies. Overall, Perfumania promises savings of as much as 70 percent, and on the most popular brands discounts of 20–25 percent. The problem is, you can't always get what you want.

An ounce of Chanel No. 5? They're out of stock. But they did have Chanel's Coco 3.3 oz. eau de parfum at $69, compared to the $110 retail price. In another case, when a specific fragrance and size were requested, I was told it was only available in a package along with the men's fragrance. But I persevered. After calling four other locations, I found the 1.7 oz. size of Fendi eau de toilette that lists for $37 for $29.95. Perfumania will take phone orders with a major credit card and ship via UPS.

# Ray Beauty Supply

721 8th Ave., bet. 45th and 46th Sts. (212) 757-0175
Hours: Monday through Friday 9:30 AM–6 PM;
Saturday 10:30 AM–5 PM

Ray Beauty Supply is in the heart of the theater district on a sleazy stretch of Eighth Avenue, but it's worth the detour: It's a great resource for beauty supplies.

Ray carries 150 different shampoos and conditioners, 15 of them for dandruff; bargain-priced professional nail polishes and nail hardeners; all types of curling irons and hair curlers; hair coloring; hennas; perms; kits for home waxing; shelves of hair sprays; hair gels (anyone for a 5 lb. tub of Queen Helene styling gel for $6.99?); shaving products; scissors; theatrical makeup; and probably the city's best selection of hand-held hairdryers, which they also service; the Swiss-made Wigo comes with a lifetime guarantee (models range from $60-$80). The fun of shopping here is that there are dozens of brands you can enjoy experimenting with. Ray delivers in Manhattan for $15, and will UPS or Fed Ex anywhere.

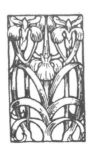

## Revlon Employee Store
767 Fifth Ave., bet. 58th and 59th Sts.  (212) 486-8857
Hours: Monday through Friday 11 AM–5:20 PM

Take the escalator down one floor below lobby level in the GM building and follow the signs to the small, one-room store for some of the cheapest buys around on beauty supplies. You never know what you'll find, but if you're a bargain hunter, this is paradise. There are manicure implements starting at less than $1; jumbo plastic bottles of Flex shampoo for $1.75; nail polish; Charles of the Ritz creams; Bill Blass fragrance; Borghese products; Opium eau de toilette; Ultima II oil-control foundation for $9.60 in a box marked $24; inexpensive fragrance gifts; and all types of flotsam and jetsam from Revlon's many divisions. All sales are final.

## Ricky's (Original Store)
718 Broadway (off Washington Pl.)  (212) 979-5232
Hours: Monday through Thursday 8 AM–11 PM;
Friday, Saturday, Sunday 8 AM–12 PM
OTHER LOCATIONS, CALL FOR HOURS:
590 Broadway bet. Houston and Prince Sts.  (212) 226-5552
44 E. 8th St. bet. Broadway and University Pl.  (212) 254-5247
466 Sixth Ave. bet. 11th and 12th Sts.  (212) 924-3401
180 Third Ave. at 17th St.  (212) 228-4485
501 Second Ave. at 28th St.  (212) 679-5435
608 Columbus Ave. bet. 89th and 90th Sts.  (212) 769-1050
1675 Third Ave. bet. 93rd and 94th Sts.  (212) 348-7400

Ricky's (Original Store) fits right in on a strip of Broadway dotted with vintage clothing stores and lots of downtown flavor. It's a spot known to models (Naomi Campbell, Lauren Hutton), actresses (Jamie Lee Curtis), makeup artists, and the Soho crowd as a fun place to shop for beauty products and low-priced beauty paraphernalia that you won't find in your neighborhood drugstore.

The colored plastic rollers that models and hairdressers use (and that we all curled our hair with and slept uncomfortably on 30 years ago) are here by the zillions along with the bobby pins and hair clips to go with them. Ricky's also has the best selection of nail files in town as well as false eyelashes; empty plastic containers for holding makeup; aluminum travel containers colored silver, gold, or made of blue glass, $2–$4; baskets and baskets of hair brushes and combs; all types of makeup puffs and sponges (Bobbi Brown buys hers here); every type of soap you can imagine, including "Chocolate Love A Lot" soap, $3.99; chic makeup bags—most in black, white or silver— that come in patent, nylon, or mesh and that you can use as evening bags (none higher than $40, and most a lot less); Erno Laszlo skincare products at half of uptown prices; and Ricky's own makeup line—Mattese—that offers the products similar to Lancôme and M.A.C. at about half the price.)

For the best of Ricky's come down to the original store at 718 Broadway; you won't find nearly as much stock or selection of unusual stuff at the other shops.

# United Beauty Products

49 W. 46th St. (212) 719-2324

Hours: Monday, Tuesday, Wednesday, Friday 9:30 AM–5:45 PM;
Thursday 9:30 AM–6:15 PM

Of course you'll find a great variety of reasonably priced shampoos,
professional hairdryers, Denman hairbrushes, nail products, and the
usual beauty supply offerings in this midtown beauty supply house.
But the real draw—and 50 percent of the business—is hair-coloring
products, and the most popular is the Miss Clairol line. United supplies products to lots of top hair salons—The Spot, Oribe, and
Roger Thompson, to name just a few—so it's worth a stop if you're
in search of a shade that you can't find in your local drugstore. In
addition to Clairol, United carries hair-color lines made by Indola
(an international line owned by Alberto Culver), L'Oréal, Revlon,
and Wella.

# Zitomer

969 Madison Ave., bet. 76th and 77th Sts. (212) 737-5560
Hours: Monday through Friday 9 AM–8 PM; Saturday 9 AM–7 PM;
Sundays and holidays 10 AM–6 PM

This posh Upper East Side pharmacy prides itself on having it all: cosmetics, hair accessories, fragrances, makeup mirrors, hats, scarves, underwear, costume jewelry, candles, electronics, even candy, videos, toys, and children's clothes.

No bargains here, but the wealth of novel beauty items, in addition to all the staples, makes it well worth the detour. It carries the hard-to-find Denman hairbrushes; tiny fold-up reading glasses, $20; a vibrating hairbrush; a fold-up eyelash curler; a fabulous Koh-I-Noor wooden wide-tooth detangling comb, $22; a tanning hat with a polymer visor that screens out 96 percent of the burning UVA rays and still allows for tanning, $75; bath oils from Canada by Pact; handmade Parisian Diptyque fragrance candles; the French LeClerc face powders; Tweezerman products; Comptoir Sud Pacifique, the French fragrances, body creams, shampoos, and bath products made with comestible essences as the basis for the scents; and homeopathic remedies for whatever ails you.

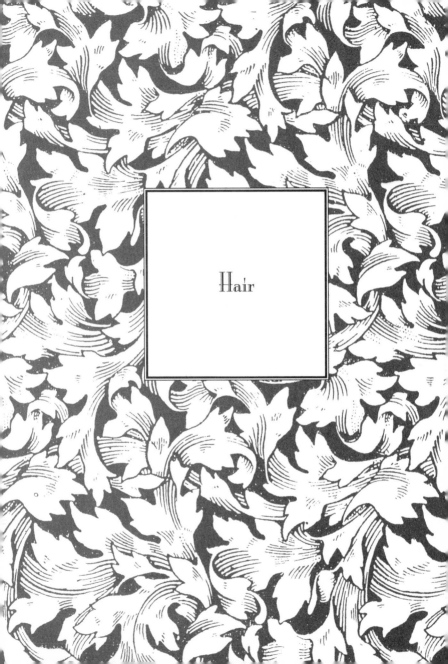

Hair

# Astor Place Hair Designers

2 Astor Place  (212) 475-9854

Hours: Monday through Saturday 8 AM–8 PM; Sunday 9 AM–6 PM

This East Village hair emporium is a hybrid of funky hair salon and macho barbershop. There are three levels, all lit by ghastly fluorescent bulbs. Floors are strewn with hair, and the mirrored work stations are surrounded by taped-up pictures of clients and hairdos. That said, this is a place that performs. No matter what your look, or how bizarre your vision, one of the 88 full-timers can do it, do it well, and do it cheaply. Haircuts start at $10 and don't go much higher unless you want your hair buzzed off except for the letters of a close friend's name, Go Knicks, or maybe the U.S. map—crew cut length—decorating the back of your skull. Those cost $25–$50.

Astor Place also does color, $25 and up; straightening, $35 and up; "Hi-Lites" (I swear the sign says that), $50 and up; manicures, and waxing. Sundays and holidays all services are $2 more.

# Jean Louis David

QUICK SERVICE

367-369 Madison Ave. at 46th St. (212) 808-9117

1385 Broadway at 38th St. (212) 869-6250

1180 Ave. of the Americas at 46th St. (212) 944-7380

303 Park Ave. South at 23rd St. (212) 260-3628

2111 Broadway at 73rd St. (212) 721-6684

783 Lexington Ave. at 61st St. (212) 838-7490

For information: (212) 808-9117

Hours: Monday, Tuesday, Wednesday, Friday,

Saturday 10 AM–7 PM; Thursday 10 AM–8 PM

Not only can you walk into these salons on the spur of the moment, but you won't have to mortgage your home to pay the bill.

Prices start at $16.50 for a shampoo and cut. Single-process haircoloring or highlighting, $47.50. Shampoo, haircut, and single process or highlighting, $58. There are 20 percent discounts for clients under age 20 as well as for those who have weekly services.

Caveat emptor: Service can be uneven. You may get a great cut one time, but not another, so if you find a stylist you like book him or her ahead for your next appointment.

# Bruno Demetrio

FREDERIC FEKKAI BEAUTY CENTER (see also p. 46, and p. 114)
Bergdorf Goodman  1 W. 57th St., 7th floor  (212) 753-9500
Hours: Tuesday, Wednesday, Friday, Saturday 9 AM–6 PM;
Thursday 9 AM–7:30 PM

Demetrio's skills have long been known to those on the New York beauty scene. He ran his own successful shop—Bruno LeSalon—for 22 years. But he closed the salon in 1994 and since then he's been doing what he does best: giving expert haircuts. In just 10 or 15 minutes, Demetrio does natural, easy-to-manage styles, no matter what the length or type of hair. The acid test of his cuts? They look good long after you leave the salon. Haircuts, $110.

TO SAVE MONEY: Demetrio oversees training sessions every Tuesday evening at 7 pm. Cuts, $25. Call for appointments.

# Sonia Gemayel

GEMAYEL SALON
2030 Broadway at 70th St.  (212) 787-5555
Hours: Monday through Friday 9 AM–7:30 PM; Saturday 9 AM–6 PM

Lebanese-born Sonia Gemayel and her husband, Said, run a full-service salon, but regulars come to her for her trendy, affordable cuts. Although there's no typical Gemayel look, she does lots of feminine styles—some sleek flips—and the kind of hair, Gemayel says with a laugh, "you see on *Melrose Place.*"

Cuts for women, $60 and up; for men, $50.

# Cohl Katz

MCM

18 W. 23rd St., 5th floor  (212) 366-5757

Hours: Monday through Friday 10 AM–6:30 PM

Cohl, as everyone calls her, was one of the three principals of this small, trendy salon, but she sold her interest to her two partners and now divides her time between cutting hair in the salon and doing editorial work. She trained with Vidal Sassoon in London and San Francisco, and has been cutting hair for 14 years.

What's she good at? Everything. Cohl is as comfortable doing short precision cuts as layering longer hair. But if you just want one-quarter inch trimmed off, that's fine, too.

"I'm not cutting hair to do the haircut of the moment or to show people how creative I can be," says Cohl. "I want clients to feel good about how they look."

Whatever the cut, it should have weight, proportion, and be versatile enough to be worn in at least two other styles, she says. Cohl also does makeup.

Women's cuts, $100; men's cuts, $80.

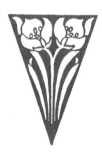

## Kim Lepine

673 Madison Ave., corner of 61st St. (212) 355-4247
Hours: Monday, Tuesday, Friday, Saturday 9 AM–5 PM;
Wednesday and Thursday, 9 AM–7 PM

Kim Lepine (pronounced le-PEEN) made her reputation as an expert haircutter during her 24-year stint as La Coupe's international art director. In mid-1994 she flew La Coupe and opened her own airy, two-story salon bearing her name. Models on the way up go to Lepine, as does a slew of women already there.

"Women don't give themselves enough style," says Lepine. "Sometimes just a small change can make a big difference." She charges a hefty $175 for a haircut, but if that's too steep she'll have one of her stylists (rates starting at $60) do the cut she recommends.

TO SAVE MONEY: Tuesday night is training night for cutting and coloring. It begins at 5:30 pm. No appointment is necessary. Candidates are picked on the basis of what the assistants need to learn. Cuts, $10–$15; color, $20–$40.

## Burton Machen

PETER COPPOLA SALON  (see also p. 45)
746 Madison Ave., bet. 64th and 65th Sts., 2nd floor  (212) 988-9404
Hours: Monday 9 AM–5 PM; Tuesday, Friday 9 AM–7 PM;
Wednesday, Saturday 9 AM–6 PM;  Thursday 9 AM–7:30 PM

"I love sexy, natural hair," says Machen. "I don't like hairdos. I don't think they're very practical."

Basic training for 24-year-old Machen was at Frederic Fekkai, and he's learned well. Soft, natural hair that falls beautifully into place is what Machen can turn out in just 20 minutes. His haircuts are all about proportion, and just as soon as he cuts it perfectly, and blows it out methodically, he goes back and has fun messing it up — perfectly.

Haircuts for women, $125; haircuts for men, $100.


## Harold Melvin

HAROLD MELVIN BEAUTY SALON
137 W. 72nd St. (212) 724-7700
Hours: Tuesday through Saturday 10 AM–10 PM

Melvin is a seasoned pro, and has run this unassuming West side salon for 21 years. His name is well known among African-American celebrities—Ruby Dee, Diahann Carroll and Harry Belafonte are clients—and he has spent much of his career working on movie sets and doing editorial work. These days he prefers a low-key schedule, and is spending more time in the salon. Aside from his basic talent—cutting—Melvin prides himself on hair care.

During a shampoo, Melvin likes to gently scrub the scalp with a brush. To keep the hair healthy, rinse thoroughly, he says. Use a conditioner after at least every other shampoo.

Haircut: $10–$20; perms, $75–$80; straightening, $60–$75; full head of braids: $175–$450 (Farrah Fawcett Majors came here for braids).

## Anita Michael

TERZETTO SALON

843 Lexington Ave., bet. 64th and 65th Sts.  (212) 717-4339

Hours: Tuesday 12:15 PM–7 PM; Wednesday 8:30 AM–5:30 PM;

Thursday 10:45 AM–6:15 PM; Friday 8:30 AM–5:30 PM;

Saturday 11 AM–4 PM

Michael has a faithful coterie of clients who have moved with her from Penta Hair Design to Pentomo and most recently to Terzetto. After a warm greeting to a client, her opening words are usually "talk to me." Michael is a listener who will suggest, never push. This is a comfortable place, not a hot spot where you'll see Ivana and Cindy, and that's its appeal. Michael's good, dependable, and ready to please. And her prices won't break the bank. Haircuts, $65.

## Lois Pisani

PIERRE MICHEL AT TRUMP TOWER (see also p. 77)

725 Fifth Ave., bet. 56th and 57th Sts.

(212) 593-1460 / (212) 753-3995 / (212) 757-5175

Pisani's hours: Tuesday, Wednesday and Friday 10 AM–5 PM;

Thursday 11 AM-7 PM; every other Saturday 11 AM-3 PM.

Devotees of Pisani's work call her a pro at cutting curly hair, but she just laughs when she hears that: "If you can cut hair, you can cut any kind of hair," And she does. And her clients return faithfully to her year after year because, as one says, she never fails.

"I do whatever makes clients happy," says Pisani. But whatever the style, "the hair should look as good from the sides and the back as from the front. I look at the total person, head and body, not a person's age. I hate age."

Haircuts for women, $75; for men, $55. If you want a colorist in the same salon, ask for Theresa Heimgartner.

## Laara Raynier
ANGELA COSMAI SALON (see also p. 45)
16 W. 55th St. (212) 541-5820
Hours: By appointment, Tuesday through Saturday

"I'm not one of those hairdressers who will sit and listen to a client tell me exactly what to do," says London-born Raynier. "I do my best when I can do whatever I want." Doing whatever she wants translates to feminine cuts with clean, carefully sculpted shapes. "I do brilliant bobs," Raynier says, with charming immodesty.

Haircuts, $85–$100.

# Vincent Roppatte

VINCENT AT SAKS (see also p. 120)
Saks Fifth Avenue
611 Fifth Ave., bet. 49th and 50th Sts. (212) 940-4069
Hours: Monday through Friday 6:30 AM-9 PM

Vincent Roppatte is an institution. He's been making celebrities and mere mortals look their best since he was 17 and won the world competition for hairdressers. He traveled with both Judy Garland and Marlene Dietrich, did Grace Kelly's hair, has done Princess Caroline's, and more recently gave Diane Sawyer her shorter cut and subtle highlights. But whether doing a celebrity or ordinary person, Roppatte aims to make the cut fit a woman's face, her hair type, and her lifestyle. He's also an expert on makeup, clothes, and accessories.

In spite of TV work, Roppatte is in the salon from the wee hours of the morning until after dinner. But be prepared to wait about a month for an appointment if you're a new client.

Haircuts, $125; highlights, $250-$300.

# Supercuts

For nearest location, call 1-800-55 SUPER
Hours: Seven days. Call for various salon hours.

This California-based company has been in business for 20 years, but in 1994-1995 alone, eight salons opened in New York. Blink and there will be several more—the company has big plans for expansion. The appeal of these clean, contemporary salons is the low price and the generally favorable reviews. Cuts are $12.75, with a shampoo, $15.75. A shampoo alone is $4. You can't book an appointment ahead of time, but you can call ahead and they'll tell you how long the wait will be. And count on a wait, unless you're the first in line when the doors open.

## Jeffrey Woodley

469 W. 57th St. (212) 246-0494
Hours: Tuesday, Wednesday, Friday, Saturday, 9 AM–5 PM;
Thursday 11 AM–7 PM

You've seen Woodley's work if you read magazines, watch videos, and go to the movies. He's done the hair of African-American celebrities such as Diahann Carroll, Whitney Houston, and Anita Baker, and he's known for making women look—in a word, glamorous. (He swears by Phytojoba shampoo and Rene Furterer Karite Creme Revitalisante conditioner.) When Woodley's not on the road, he works out of his duplex salon just a few blocks west of Carnegie Hall.

Aside from hairstyling, Woodley is also known for making wigs. He's the designer for "It's a Wig," and makes good-looking synthetic wigs for clients—of Kanekalon fiber—at astonishing low prices ($150-$200).

Want your makeup done? Woodley's partner, Eric Spearman, is fabulous.

# Color Czars

## Michael Brimhall

GIL GAMLIELI BEAUTY GROUP
820 Madison Ave., bet. 68th and 69th Sts. (212) 570-2455
Hours: Tuesday, Friday, Saturday 9 AM–6 PM;
Wednesday, Thursday 9 AM–8 PM

Brimhall's mentor was Constance Harnett, the queen of color at Frederic Fekkai. Now a graduate with honors, he has a loyal and fast-growing list of clients, who rave about his delicate hair-painting technique. The result: beautiful, natural-looking hair. Just ask Cindy Crawford or Elle McPherson. Need a haircut too? Have Gil Gamlieli cut your hair first. He and Brimhall are a top team.

Highlights, $250 and up; single process, $85 and up.

TO SAVE MONEY: Try the training classes that Brimhall teaches on Tuesday morning from 9 to 10. Haircut, single-process coloring, or highlights, $20. Call for an appointment.

# Clairol Product Evaluation Salon

345 Park Ave., bet. 51st and 52nd Sts. Center Lobby  (212) 546-2701
Interview hours: Monday through Friday 9:30 AM–11 AM,
or 1:30 PM–4 PM

Just because haircoloring prices at top salons are going through the roof doesn't mean that those *sans l'argent* can't have their hair done by the pros. From Monday to Friday this in-house salon in the Clairol building offers free hair-coloring services as a way to test out new products, shades, and formulas.

Don't worry about coming away with hair like a Barbie doll. "We want people to be happy," says a Clairol spokesman. Bottom line: they won't turn a gorgeous brunette into a platinum blonde. They'll go with your particular coloring and find a color or product that will work on you. Everyone is told what products have been used and how to use them at home. And if you're thrilled with the results, you can come back.

Services are done all day by appointment. Only requirements: You must be 18 years of age or older and show up for an interview first.

# Angela Cosmai

ANGELA COSMAI SALON (see also p.40)

16 W. 55th St., 2nd floor  (212) 541-5820

Hours: Tuesday through Friday 10 AM–6 PM; one Saturday a month

Cosmai's forte is corrective color. Translation: she can fix haircoloring disasters. Case in point: It was Cosmai who corrected  Melanie Griffith's wild mane after "Working Girl."

"A lot of women go overboard when it comes to haircoloring," says Cosmai. "They don't look as good as they could because they do too much." Her approach, instead, is to create believable color, with highlights that whisper rather than shout. Every eight weeks she flies to L.A. to do her regulars, and every six weeks she heads south to do Florida clients.

Single process, $100; full-head highlights, $400; half-head, $250.

TO SAVE MONEY: Cosmai oversees training sessions on Wednesday nights from 5 PM–7:30 PM. Cost, $25–$40. Call for an appointment.

# Sharon Dorram

PETER COPPOLA SALON (see also p. 37)

746 Madison Ave., bet. 64th and 65th Sts., 2nd floor  (212) 988-9404

Hours: Tuesday through Friday 8:30 AM–7 PM; alternating Saturdays 8:30 AM–7 PM

Sharon Dorram trained at La Coupe when Louis Licari headed the color department, and her polished skills are known about town.

Natural yet opulent color is her signature, with brightness around the face. "I go back to the hair color you had when you were younger, and nine out of ten times that means lighter," says Dorram. She also opts for low-maintenance color, so if you don't have much gray she'll just do highlights instead of single process and highlights. To maintain color between salon visits, Dorram recommends Phyto neutral shampoo.

Single process, $100; highlights, $150 to $300.

## Constance Harnett

FREDERIC FEKKAI BEAUTY CENTER (see also pp. 35, 114)
Bergdorf Goodman  1 W. 57th St., 7th floor  (212) 753-9500
Harnett's hours: Monday through Friday 8 AM-5 PM

Haircolorists around the country speak of Constance Harnett, the "Queen of Haircolor," in hushed, reverent tones, and her client list reads like a Who's Who of America's best-looking women. Over the course of a career spanning close to 30 years, she has taught many professionals the delicate hair-painting techniques she learned in Paris.

Harnett's keen sense of color goes back to her training in product development at Revlon in the late 1960s, and later her stint as color director for the former salon operator, Glemby International. These days it doesn't take her more than a glance to detect sloppy technique or the wrong hues.

Single process, $110; single process with some hair-painting, $140–$150; color and highlighting, $250–$275; whole head highlighting, $250–$300.

TO SAVE MONEY: Look for Harnett at the teaching classes, Tuesday nights at six. Single-process color or highlights, $30. Cutting is not done the same week as color. Call for an appointment.

## Brad Johns

ORIBE SALON
691 Fifth Ave., bet. 54th and 55th Sts., 10th floor  (212) 319-3910
Hours: Wednesday through Saturday 8:30 AM–4:30 PM

Although it is housed on the 10th floor of Elizabeth Arden, the Oribe salon is a far cry from the sedate Red Door world around it. It's ornate, with Venetian mirrors, crystal chandeliers, gilded seats, and terrific, gutsy hair services: case in point, Brad Johns, color director.

If your look is *au naturel,* Johns is not for you. He doesn't think your hair color should be subtle. His color turns heads—it's bold and vibrant. He copies the way children's hair color looks at the beach, he says, using mixtures of caramel, toffee, nutmeg, cinnamon, and warm reddish golds. "Ashy colors don't look good," says Johns.

His philosophy: "Hair color should complement the eyes first, the skin second, and the season third." Typically, he applies the most color—chunks of highlights—at the front of the face.

Single process, $100; highlights, $250.

# Louis Licari

LOUIS LICARI COLOR GROUP

797 Madison Avenue, 2nd floor  (212) 517-8084

Hours: For Licari, Monday through Friday, by appointment.

Salon open Monday through Saturday from 7:30 AM.

Closing times vary; call for hours.

Licari's clients coming in for color look better than the ones walking out of other salons. "King of Color" Licari, a consultant to Clairol and a makeover magician, has a steady following of high-powered women who start believing those natural-looking highlights are really their own.

His philosophy is minimal color for maximum effect, and he knows how to accent a wave, warm up your skin tone, and use haircolor as a cosmetic.

Licari's schedule is booked tight, and he spends every third week in his L.A. salon—but if you're willing to sit tight till an appointment opens up, you can bet he'll turn you into a much better-looking version of yourself. If you can't or won't wait, you can book an appointment on short notice with one of his nine colorists.

Single process, $100; highlights, $300–$400; single process plus highlights, $300-$400. Rates with other colorists: Single process, $55–$75; highlights, $125–$200; single process plus highlights, $130–$225.

TO SAVE MONEY: Color and cut classes are Wednesday nights (or sometimes Tuesdays) from 6 to 10:30. Single process, $15.60; highlights, $26; single process plus highlights, $30; perms, $26 (scheduled every three to four months); cuts, $15.60. Classes are booked one month in advance. Call on Tuesday afternoon beween 2:00 and 4:00 and ask for an appointment for either color or cutting class night.

## Donna McNally

BRIAN PICKSTON HAIR SPA
24 E. 22nd St. (212) 228-4422
Hours: Wednesday through Friday 11 AM–8 PM; Saturday 9 AM–6 PM

McNally aquired much of her technical expertise while working as an assistant to salon operator and Redken consultant Beth Minardi. McNally was a top student; She has a sharp eye for picking the right hair color, keying it to eye and skin color. These days she works downtown, and over the past few years has developed her own diverse client following, including a sprinkling of Ford models and some graying men who'd prefer not to be.

Single process, $60; highlights from $90–$175.

# Beth Minardi

MINARDI SALON (see also p. 72)
29 E. 61st St., 5th floor  (212) 308-1711
Hours: Monday, Tuesday, Saturday 9 AM–5 PM;
Wednesday, Thursday, Friday 9 AM–8 PM (last appointment)

Never mind natural; when Minardi, a consultant to Redken, colors hair she makes it look shiny and better than natural. She's one of the few colorists who believes in double processing when one wants truly pale, pastel blond hair.

Most of Minardi's clients want highlights, however, and she has developed a technique known as multi-directional highlighting, which means hair is wrapped in two separate directions, each with different colors. The tic-tac-toe board effect gives the hair a more complex blend of color, which is closer to nature—á la client Sara Jessica Parker—than the striped effect many women suffer after highlighting.

Single-process color and glaze, $88; double-process color change from $150; highlights from $220. Minardi also custom-blends color shampoos for between-salon visits ($15) and will recommend colorists around the country for clients who travel.

TO SAVE MONEY: Training classes for color and cutting are on Tuesdays at 4 pm. Color and cut each $15. Call for an appointment.

# Brian Murphy

THE SPOT

521 Madison Ave. bet. 53rd and 54th Sts., 4th floor  (212) 688-4450

Hours: Monday through Saturday 8:30 AM–8 PM

Careful, simple, less-is-more haircoloring is Brian Murphy's signature. He's not one to be flamboyant, heavy-handed with color, or consumed by the latest trends. And if he's asked to make a dramatic color change, he may well first test the product on a strand of the client's hair before he applies it all over the head, to see if the chemistry works. Murphy takes his time and listens to what his clients want.

Single process, $70; full-head highlights, $170; half-head, $120.

TO SAVE MONEY: Training night is Wednesday at 5:45 PM. Color and cut each $15. Call for an appointment.

## The Philip Kingsley Trichological Clinic

16 E. 53rd St. (212) 753-9600 / 1-800-745-1653
Hours: Monday, Tuesday, Wednesday, Friday 9 AM–4:15 PM;
Thursday 9 AM–6:30 PM; Saturday 9 AM–3:15 PM

Kingsley has been dealing with all sorts of hair problems for 35 years through his London clinic and, since 1977, in New York. A visit begins with an analysis and case history, nutrition advice, and some discussion of hair care ($150 by Kingsley, $100 by another trichologist). If a medical problem is suspected, a client may be asked to go for blood work. Kingsley works with physicians at Mount Sinai hospital.

After the consultation comes treatment: application of a scalp potion and hair conditioner, scalp massage, infrared lamps to help products penetrate, shampoo, a second conditioner, and scalp tonic. Individual treatments, $57.50, cheaper if purchased in a series of five or more.

Kingsley markets his own product line made on the premises— 6.7 ozs. of shampoo or conditioner, $12; 4.2 ozs. of intensive antidandruff treatment, $20.

TO SAVE MONEY: The $25 phone consultation. Describe your problems, fill out a questionnaire, send it back, and have the appropriate products sent to you. They're extra, of course.

# J.F. Lazartigue Diagnostic and Advisory Hair Care Center

764 Madison Ave., bet. 65th and 66th Sts. (212) 288-2250
Hours: Monday through Saturday 10 AM–6 PM

The treatment at this gleaming-white hair-care center does for your hair and scalp what posh skin-care salons do for your face and body. You get shampooed, conditioned, pampered, soothed, and treated to one of the best head, neck, upper-back and upper-arm massages in town. You emerge feeling calm, with a head of hair that has never looked shinier or bouncier. Sound good? Go for it. Just prepare to pay big bucks. And if you're interested in buying the products, you're talking investment.

The one and three-quarter hour treatment begins with a technician parting your hair, brushing it, and talking to you about hair care, diet, and lifestyle. Then a hair is plucked from your scalp and examined under a microscope that magnifies the hair and bulb 180 times. A diagnosis is made; an appropriate treatment begins.

One regimen for a healthy scalp: Cleansing the scalp with propolis jelly, applying orange-colored carrot conditioner, mild steaming for 15 minutes, a shampoo followed by a conditioner combed through and left on for ten minutes, a fab massage, hairstyling, and blow-dry. The tab, $150.

Want to continue the regimen at home? My prescription list added up to a whopping $219.

## Adding On:
## Wigs & Hair Extensions

## Jacques Darcel
50 W. 57th St. (212) 753-7576
Hours: Monday through Saturday 10 AM–6 PM

Sixty percent of this midtown wig store's clients suffer from hair loss, and the wig is a necessity rather than a fashion accessory. Darcel offers a wide variety of wigs, which are made at the company's factories in Thailand, the Philippines, and Japan. Synthetic wigs start at $225; human-hair wigs start at $1800; and a combination of hand-tied wigs made of half human and half synthetic hair range from $695 to $1,200. Wigs can be tried in private fitting booths.

The salon cuts, styles, and cleans wigs. To discourage browsers, there is an initial $35 consultation fee, applicable toward the price.

## Andre J. Davis
230 W. 55th St. (212) 757-4415
Hours: Monday through Saturday, by appointment

Davis's expertise at weaving in individual sections of human hair is more and more in demand these days. His clients are not only models, celebrities, and the theatre crowd but also those with hair loss.

Hair extensions are individual sections of human hair. Each section, or weft, is attached by weaving it into a very fine braid, that runs horizontally along the scalp. Extensions are far more comfortable to wear than a wig because they're light, cool, and don't cover the scalp. They're also generally indistinguishable from one's own hair—even if there's little of it. Davis says that even when hair loss is extensive he can help. Consultations are free.

Costs add up, however. Extensions range from $200 to about $700 for a full head of human European hair. They can be left in as long as three-and-a-half to four months, but as hair grows they must be carefully removed and replaced with new ones. Unless Davis has a perfect color match in stock, special orders take one week.

## Bob Kelly Wig Creations
151 W. 46th St. (212) 819-0030 / 1-800-339-4863
Hours: Monday through Friday 7:30 AM–2 PM

Bob Kelly is a respected name in the field, widely known for his custom wigs for Broadway as well as his professional makeup line. But Kelly also makes wigs, hair extensions, and hair pieces for people with hair loss, and you can save money here, since his wigs sell for more at other salons.

Custom human-hair wigs start at $1,500 and take two to three weeks to make. Hair extensions cost about $350 for a full head. Kelly doesn't make synthetic wigs, but recommends places such as It's a Wig (36 W. 37th St., 212-594-6111) and W & Y Chung Traders (1225

Broadway, at 30th St., 212-683-2767). Consultations are free. Private customers interested in custom wigs should call Joe for an appointment.

## Ruth L. Weintraub Co. Inc.

CUSTOM WIGS AND HAIRPIECES
420 Madison Ave., bet. 48th and 49th Sts., 4th floor  (212) 838-1333
Hours: Monday through Friday 10 AM-5 PM

Weintraub has a long track record in the business, and a sympatico attitude. Her specialty is custom-made wigs from either human hair —$2,200 and up—or synthetic material. Although synthetic hair is cheaper, these "sport models" are more labor-intensive and thus more expensive, says Weintraub. Prices start at $2,500, but on the plus side, synthetic wigs are easier to care for and last longer. It takes three fittings over three weeks to make a custom wig.

Weintraub also sells some "customized wigs." These are ready-made wigs that can be adjusted somewhat to fit head size. Customized human-hair wigs start at $1,200; customized synthetics start at $500.

Free catalog and literature are available. Consultations are free.

# Taking It Off:
## Electrolysis

CAVEAT EMPTOR: There are no licensing requirements for electrologists in New York State. Anyone can call him or herself an electrologist. Following is a sampling of well-trained professionals:

## Cynthia Cordero
252 W. 79th St. (212) 724-5171
Hours: By appointment, Tuesday, Wednesday, Thursday
10 AM–7:30 PM; alternate Saturdays 10 AM–4 PM

Cordero, who received her training with Lucy Peters, has been practicing for 15 years. She uses the short-wave method and the insulated bulbous probe. After a free consultation, she suggests shaving the area before beginning treatment to eliminate the chance of treating dormant hairs (they'll only grow back if they're treated in this stage). Clients are told how long initial clearing will take—as few as two sessions if the area was never tweezed or waxed—and up to three months of weekly visits if it was. Then monthly maintenance visits are needed for anywhere from six to eight months.

Rates: $85 per hour; $45 per half-hour; $30 for 15 minutes.

# Dawn Electrolysis

118 E. 59th St., Suite 305  (212) 935-2918 / (212) 935-2900
Hours: By appointment, Tuesday through Friday 10 AM–7 PM;
Saturday 10 AM–5 PM

Dawn Edison works from a small, immaculate office just down the street from Bloomingdale's. She uses a short-wave electrolysis machine with the insulated bulbous probe. Most patients begin treatment with the shaving of the area to be cleaned. How long does treatment take? Six months to one year. If you're going to an electrologist and you don't see significant improvement in an area within six months, find someone else, advises Edison.

Rates: $80 per hour; $30 per half-hour; $25 for 15 minutes.

# Lucy Peters International, Ltd.

150 E. 58th St. (212) 486-9740

Hours: Monday through Friday 9 AM–7 PM; Saturday 9 AM–5 PM

Lucy Peters International is probably the gold standard in electrolysis treatment. There are seven offices around the country, including one in Philadelphia at the University City Science Center and another at Duke University Medical Center.

Ms. Peters has long been a proponent of the insulated bulbous probe, which directs the flow of electricity to the probe's tip, providing current to destroy hair growth at its source, without damaging surrounding skin. The probe is also safer, she claims, because it slips easily into hair follicles and can't pierce surrounding skin. All Peter's technicians are company trained.

Clients are told how many visits treatment will take. All methods of hair removal except shaving are stopped so that the operator can see which hairs regrow—only hairs in the growing stage can be effectively treated.

Rates: $100 per hour; for two or more consecutive hours, $115 per hour; $65 per half-hour or less.

# Saving Face

## Skin Care & Makeup

# Mario Badescu Inc. Skin Care

320 E. 52nd St. (212) 758-1065

Hours: Monday, Tuesday, Thursday, Friday 10 AM–5 PM;
Wednesday 11 AM–7 PM; Saturday 9 AM–5 PM

Two chemists with medical backgrounds, the late Mario Badescu and
Benone Genesco, started this salon 28 years ago. They never adver-
tised. Now Genesco runs the salon with his chemist wife; business is
booming; and it's all due to word of mouth and favorable press.

The Badescu philosophy is simple: go with nature. It calls for
gentle cleansing and moisturizing with natural products, and as few
harsh chemicals as possible—mineral oil is anathema. Sound modern? It is, but at Badescu things haven't changed much in almost
three decades.

Aside from the $55 facials done by European-trained estheti-
cians, regulars swear by the products, based on heavy doses of fresh
fruits whipped up daily on the premises. Fruit acids, so popular in
recent years, have been a staple of the salon's minimally preserved
products made from strawberries, papaya, and oranges. Other natural helpers in the product line: cucumber, bee pollen, aloe, chamomile,
seaweed, olive oil, and even caviar. Products range in price from
about $9 to $20. Other services: electrolysis, waxing, bleaching,
manicures, and pedicures.

## Christiana & Carmen Beauty Center
128 Central Park South at 59th St.  (212) 757-5811
Hours: Monday through Saturday 8:30 AM–7 PM

This small skin-care salon on Central Park South rubs shoulders
with some of the city's best hotels. It's a spot that has attracted out-
of-towners as well as local celebrities (Candice Bergen's a neighbor
and client) for most of its 17 years. Run by Christiana Salvetiu (her
mother Carmen is retired), the salon offers facials, massage, makeup,
manicures, and pedicures. For relaxing massages, Christiana is the
one. If your body needs revving up, ask for Kaiko, the Shiatsu spe-
cialist. Massage, $65 for 45 minutes with Christiana, or one hour
with her associates. Facials, $65; manicures, $15; pedicures, $31;
makeup application, $40; application with lesson included, $48.

## Diane Young Anti-Aging Skin Care Salon
38 E. 57th St., 8th floor  (212) 753-1200
Hours: Monday through Thursday 10 AM–8 PM;
Friday 10 AM–6 PM; Saturday 9 AM–5 PM

Diane Young has run a skin-care salon for 12 years, but more recently has zeroed in on antiaging help. Her arsenal of aids includes products made with papaya and pineapple enzymes, which dissolve dead
cells and speed up cell turnover; and treatments such as the "Years
Younger Facial" to smooth lines and wrinkles, $85; a "Rapid
Exfoliation Procedure, $65; and one of the newest salon offerings, the
"Oxygen Intensive Treatment," $65.

The latter doesn't involve deep breathing: A hydrogen peroxide, vitamin, and mineral potion is sprayed on your face. It breaks down on the skin, Young explains, delivering oxygen and water. She swears that it leaves her own skin baby-soft, but admits the benefits aren't as dramatic for everyone.

Other offerings: massage, waxing, manicures, pedicures, and makeup lessons. In addition to skin-care products, Young markets her own color cosmetics, and gives personal consultations, $100.

# Jennifer Dunn, R.N.
SKIN CARE/ELECTROLYSIS
Medical Office of Stephen Kurtin, M.D.
111 E. 71st St. (212) 772-1717
Hours: Monday and Wednesday 9:30 AM–7 PM;
every other Friday 9:30 AM–3 PM

As well as electrolysis, Dunn, a registered nurse, gives medical facials to Kurtin's patients. What's a medical facial? It's none of the "puff and fluff," as Dunn describes the types of facials given at spas and salons. No cucumber lotion on the eyes, no massage, no scented creams. Instead, a medical facial is a pore-cleansing treatment— mostly on acne patients—that generally follows the doctor's examination. It involves removing blackheads and whiteheads, draining pimples, and sometimes applying a mask. The treatment is included in the initial visit with the dermatologist, which costs $150. Follow-ups with Dunn alone are $60.

# Estela Gilboe

Home studio: (212) 410-2405
Let's Face It! 568 Broadway, corner of Prince St. (212) 219-8970
Hours: At Gilboe's studio: By appointment only,
Tuesday, Thursday, Saturday 9 AM -8 PM
At Let's Face It!: Monday 12:30–8 PM; Wednesday 11 AM–5 PM;
Friday 11 AM–5 PM

Gilboe divides her week between giving facials in her Upper East
Side studio and at Let's Face It!, a Soho salon popular with a young
downtown crowd. One facial with European-trained Gilboe is
enough to make you a lifetime subscriber.

The hour-plus is calming and therapeutic. She cleanses the skin,
massages the face, neck, upper back and arms, uses an exfoliating gel,
extracts blackheads, uses a toner, does a gentle peel, and ends with an
appropriate mask. She has a light touch and never leaves the skin
red. Gilboe also offers an expert skin cleaning treatment for
teenagers, sans massage. Other services: waxing, brow tweezing,
herbal wraps, and exfoliating body treatments.

Basic facial in her studio, $55. Basic facial at Let's Face It!, $65.

## Look Good . . . Feel Better

AMERICAN CANCER SOCIETY

19 W. 56th St. (212) 586-8700

Hours: Once a month, usually the third Monday, 5 PM–7:30 PM

These free monthly makeover sessions supported by the American Cancer Society, the Cosmetic, Toiletry, and Fragrance Association, and the National Cosmetology Association are designed to help improve the appearance and boost the spirits of women undergoing chemotherapy or radiation.

Makeup artists teach classes of approximately ten the how-to's of skin care and makeup application—with particular tips for camouflaging treatment side-effects, such as eyelash and eyebrow loss. Participants are given makeup to take home, free of charge, and if they need wigs, those are available too. Women must call and register first and give the name of their oncologist.

## Trish McEvoy

800 Fifth Ave. at 61st St., Suite 401 (212) 758-7790

To order makeup 1-800-431-4306

Hours: Monday through Friday 7:30 AM–7 PM; two Saturdays a month 8 AM –12:30 PM; no weekends during the summer

Makeup lessons, no-nonsense facials, and dermatology with an emphasis on cosmetic problems are all part of this skin-care practice shared by Trish McEvoy and dermatologist Ronald E. Sherman.

McEvoy recently introduced her own line of cosmetics and uses them during hour-long makeup lessons, as do five other cosmeticians. Pay close attention to what she does. She applies makeup to one side of your face—you do the other.

One of her tricks: apply eye-makeup before other products, then clean undereye area with eye makeup remover on a Q-tip. That dark dust on the Q-tip would have made your eyes look shadowy and tired, she points out.

A lesson with McEvoy costs $300, and $200 with her associates. But don't gasp. That includes a little shopping bag chock-full of all the makeup used. Brushes are extra. (They're great, but *très cher*). The foundation and the divine eye shadow base/undereye concealer—Protective Shield—have an SPF of 15. The foundation costs $35. The Protective Shield's $21. Four-color eye shadow compacts are $35.

Facials here are not the pampering kind. They take half an hour, and are only for certain conditions, such as acne. Cost (including doctor's visit, but not a sit-down consultation), $95.

## June Meyer

FACIAL DYNAMICS
129 E. 80th St. (212) 794-2961
Hours: Winter: Monday, Saturday 10 AM–6 PM;
Tuesday, Wednesday, Thursday 10 AM–10 PM;
summer: Tuesday, Wednesday, Thursday 10 AM–10 PM

Before Meyer touches your face, she asks questions: What do you use on your face? What's your history of sun exposure? Do you take vitamins? Do you smoke? And on and on. Then you change, don a shower cap, and she examines your skin. What's the facial like? It depends on your skin type and the kind of facial you prefer—heavy on the shoulder and neck massage, light on the face, etc. But the bottom line is, she'll clean your face thoroughly, remove blackheads, and leave your skin feeling velvety soft.

You can buy the products she uses (the Murad glycolic acid line, the Australian Jurlique line, especially the Deep Penetrating Cream Mask, and the Swiss Karin Herzog line), but she doesn't push them. She's just as likely to endorse inexpensive drugstore brands such as Oil of Olay, Dove, Basis soap, Moisturèl, and if you're a fan of toners, old-fashioned Witch Hazel.

A 90-minute facial, including leg, arm, and shoulder massage, $95. A two-hour treatment including back massage, $125. Meyer also does waxing. Full leg and bikini, $45.

## Elena Pociu
23 E. 67th St. (212) 717-5543
Hours: Monday through Saturday 9 AM–7 PM

The staff and clients from the upstairs Lotte Berke exercise studio are loyal fans of Pociu (pronounced po-chew), a reserved Romanian woman who runs a full-service skin-care salon. Facials are her specialty, and like other well-trained estheticians she's a proponent of a light touch and a less-is-more philosophy when it comes to products. She whips up her own macerated fruit masks on the premises and shuns many commercial products.

Want to make your own natural exfoliating product for home use? Mix one half cup bran with the yolk of one egg if your skin is dry, or the white if it's oily, and a few tablespoons of chamomile tea.

What should the acne-prone use to clean their skin? A mixture of two tablespoons of milk and six drops of lemon juice. Saturate a cotton ball and wipe the face. Rinse with a chamomile tea infusion. (Let the tea bag steep for 15 minutes. Allow the tea to cool.)

Want a natural antiseptic? Mix two parts water, boiled and cooled, with one part apple cider vinegar.

Facials, $60. One-hour massage, $60.

## Sumati Rajput

PENTOMO SALON
24 E. 64th St., 2nd floor  (212) 371-0703
Hours: Tuesday, Wednesday, Friday 9:30 AM–5 PM;
Thursday 10 AM–7 PM; Saturday 8:30 AM–3 PM

"An hour with Sumati is like a week at an ashram," says one devoted client. At the very least, the hour-long facial is a brief vacation, which takes place in a quiet room of this airy East Side townhouse, one flight up from the Pentomo hair salon.

The treatment involves cleansing, exfoliating, steaming, pore-cleaning and  disinfecting, a soothing face, neck, and back massage with aromatic oils, and finally a mask. Facials, $70.

Another specialty of the 20-year veteran is removing superfluous facial hair using an Indian technique known as threading. Excess facial hair—on brows, upper lip, the chin, or the sides of the face—

is plucked away with lightning speed by catching it between two threads that are knitted together.

"It pulls hair from the roots without pulling skin," says Rajput, "and it shapes brows better than waxing."

Full face, $35; brows, $12; upper lip, $12.


# Lia Schorr

686 Lexington Ave., bet. 56th and 57th Sts. (212) 486-9670
Hours: Monday through Friday 9 AM–8 PM;
Saturday, Sunday 9 AM–5 PM


Schorr started her skin-care salon in 1980 with $500. Today this hands-on manager oversees a full-scale operation that provides any and all beauty services—there's even a on-premises school for estheticians.

Don't be put off by Schorr's aggressive salesmanship: her staff of 18 is expert—she'd oust anyone who wasn't—and best known for facials. (Try to book with Eugyna). There's a whole menu to choose from, including deep pore cleaning, acne facials, collagen facials (don't expect miracles, as the collagen is not injected), back facials, and antistress facials. Price range, $56–$100.

TO SAVE MONEY, ask for Schorr's periodic "sales," or beauty packages. Even cheaper is the $15 45-minute facial offered between 5:30 and 8:30 PM on Mondays, Tuesdays, or Wednesdays with one of Schorr's students. Call for an appointment. Ask about other reduced-price treatments given by supervised students.

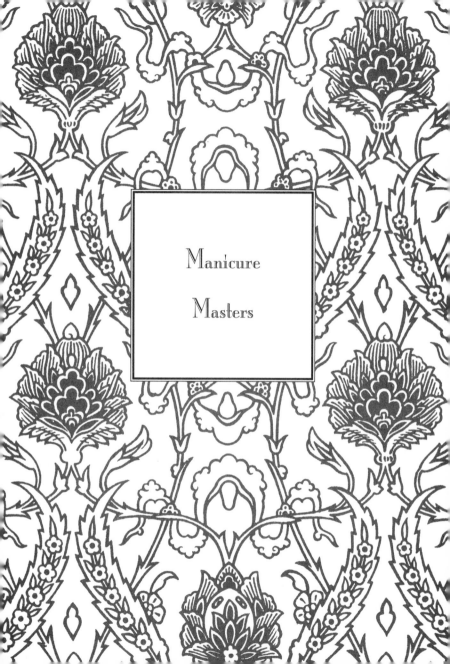

Manicure

Masters

# Lucy Bran

IRENE & LUCY
223 E. 74th St. (212) 772-0720
Hours: Tuesday through Saturday 9 AM–6 PM

Lucy Bran is literally at the feet of Upper East Side women. The small, middle-of-the-block salon she runs with her partner, Irene, is simple and unadorned, but the service is always high-quality. Bran has been practicing for almost 20 years; she does manicures and pedicures, but regulars book her a month ahead for pedicures. She keeps clients' own implement kits tucked away for them, and has been sterilizing instruments before it became law. Aside from her thorough nail-cleaning and grooming, she is known for her leg massages.

Manicures, $11; pedicures, $27. Prices are double for house calls.

# Mariana Condeescu

DESSIE & ALINA AT YOUR FINGERTIPS
309 E. 75th St. (212) 794-6588
Hours: Tuesday, Wednesday, Friday, Saturday 10 AM–7:30 PM;
Thursday 10 AM–8:30 PM

Mariana Condeescu has been giving manicures and pedicures for 25 years, and she has a regular following on the Upper East Side. Condeescu is gentle and takes her time with each client, meticulously grooming the nails with sterilized instruments, pushing back cuticles, filing nails perfectly, and applying polish so it lasts. Ask her about the latest nail booster, and except for Nailtique, she'll probably raise an eyebrow and look at you as if to say, "Don't you know better?"

Manicure, $12.50; pedicure, $25

## Donia Gonta

ELLEGEE NAIL SALON
22 E. 66th St.  (212) 472-5063
Gonta's hours: Monday through Friday 8:30 AM–6:30 PM

Gonta is one of New York's best for nail care. She's careful, thorough, and meticulous, and when she finishes your pedicure you'll feel like showing off your feet in a pair of sexy sandals. The salon is small and low-key so you avoid a hectic atmosphere. Another pro at this salon: part-owner Gabby Nigai—Barbra Streisand's manicurist when she's in town.

Manicure, $15; pedicure, $35. The salon also does waxing.

## Cornelia Lerescu/Manicurist
## Florina Radu/Pedicurist

MINARDI SALON  (see also p. 50)
29 E. 61st St., 5th floor  (212) 308-1711
Hours: Tuesday, Wednesday, Friday 10 AM–6 PM;
Thursday 10 AM–8 PM; Saturday 9 AM–5 PM

The Minardi salon is best known for haircuts and color, but nail experts Lerescu and Radu are two jewels in its crown.

For those short of time, they do manicures and pedicures simultaneously. If you have the treatments consecutively, allot a good portion of the morning or afternoon. A pedicure with Radu takes over an hour, and Lerescu makes sure your oil-painted nails and cuticles soak in warm cream long enough to absorb the moisture. To strengthen nails, she uses Nailtique as a basecoat, and finishes a manicure with a non-yellowing topcoat to keep it looking fresh.

Radu, who prefers to do pedicures, is a big fan of tea-tree oil, which she squirts into the foot bath. It's antifungal and antibacterial, and she says she has seen remarkable improvement in clients who use the oil nightly for stubborn cases of fungal infections. After the soaking, Radu tells a client "give me the good foot." That's the one she starts with. The other gets to soak longer.

After a thorough cleaning, she gives advice for at-home care: "I teach clients not to cut calluses too much, and each time they shower to use a pumice stone." Those who have corns are urged to try Dr. Scholl's toe pads to relieve pressure and prevent thickening.

Manicure, $15; pedicure, $35; house calls twice the price of a service, plus transportation.


# Barbara Mutnick

(212) 772-7486
Hours: Seven days, by appointment


The bell rings: Hello, manicure. Seven days a week, early morning to late evening, Mutnick crosses Manhattan, visiting homes, offices, and hotels doing manicures and pedicures. She carries a beeper and says that she's almost always on call. Her black bag is packed with all the essentials: lamp, sterilized tools, files, creams, polish, quick-drying top coat. All you need is a towel. Her regulars are visiting celebrities and high-powered executives who know they can beep her even on short notice and she'll show up. Between manicures, Mutnick tells clients to break open vitamin E capsules and use the oil on their nails and hands.

Manicure, $50. Pedicure, $65.


## Nails by Nina
129 E. 80th St. (212) 288-8130
Hours: Monday 12 PM–8 PM
Tuesday through Friday 8 AM–7:30 PM


On a scale of one to ten, Nina Novy is a 12. She's a soft-spoken Russian woman who's shy and self-effacing. Only in the course of a manicure or pedicure does a client realize that she's one of the most knowledgeable nail pros around.

Novy doesn't use soapy water to soak nails because it's too drying. She doesn't cut cuticles; she's largely against sculpted nails, and she avoids harmful glues or other chemicals known to trigger adverse reactions. She's also against common salon practices such as reusing paraffin for manicures and pedicures. What she does do is methodically clean and groom the nails and surrounding skin, file nails, massage hands, and neatly apply polish. Manicures take 45 minutes. In addition to manicures, $17, and pedicures, $31, Novy does waxing.

# Jonice Padilha

J. SISTERS

35 W. 57th St. (212) 750-2485 / (212) 750-0170

Hours: Tuesday, Friday, Saturday 9 AM–6 PM

Wednesday, Thursday 8:30 AM–7:30 PM (last appointment)

Five Brazilian sisters who all have first names that start with the letter J (Joyce, Jonice, Jane, Jussara, and Jocely) run this full-service salon known for its manicures and pedicures. Jonice Padilha—whose client list reads like a Who's Who in the beauty field—isn't much interested in the color of nail polish or the shape you want your nails filed. Her focus is on cuticles, and if yours have gotten ragged because of neglect, nervous nibbling, or inferior manicures, she'll come to the rescue.

While an average manicure may take 20 minutes, Jonice may spend more than an hour on the cuticles. But clients who won't let a manicurist put anything but an orange stick anywhere near the cuticles beware: Jonice doesn't take no for an answer.

Manicures, $17 and up; pedicures, $45 for the first time (count on two hours); follow-ups, $40.

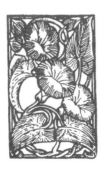

# Roxana Pintilie

WARREN TRICOMI

16 W. 57th St., 4th floor  (212) 262-8899

Hours: Monday 10 AM–6 PM; Tuesday through Saturday 8 AM–8 PM

Nail pro Roxana Pintilie, part-owner of this elegant 57th St. salon, spends part of her time on film shoots, part on cable television talking about the ABCs of manicures, and the rest in the salon, where she has taught the staff her techniques.

How do her manicures differ? Pintilie starts by massaging the hands with cream and then putting them in heated mitts to warm and soften the skin. She doesn't believe in soaking the hands in water because, she says, it's drying and can spread fungus and germs. Another Pintilie principle: never cut the cuticles. Dermatologists would agree, since the cuticles act as a natural barrier against infection. Pintilie thinks of a manicure in terms of nail hygiene rather than pure cosmetics. Thumbs up!

Other services: Hair cuts; color; scalp treatments; massage; paraffin manicures and pedicures; and hand and foot facials.

Manicure, $15–$20.

# Geta Tocaciu

PIERRE MICHEL (see also p. 39)
Trump Tower 725 Fifth Ave., bet. 56th and 57th Sts.
(212) 593-1460 / (212) 753-3995 / (212) 757-5175
Hours: Monday through Friday 9 AM–6 PM

Fourteen years ago, Tocaciu started her career in New York as a manicurist. Before that, she worked as a pediatric nurse in her native Romania. It's easy to imagine her as a health professional—she's strong, gentle, and authoritative, and you trust her instincts from the get go.

You don't have to tell her what shape to file your nails. She matches the shape to the shape of your fingers and cuticles. She's careful not to file too much from the sides of the nails because that would weaken them. And for your feet, pedicures aren't a luxury, they're a necessity, she says, especially for women who spend long hours standing.

Manicure, $20; pedicure, $40.

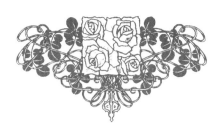

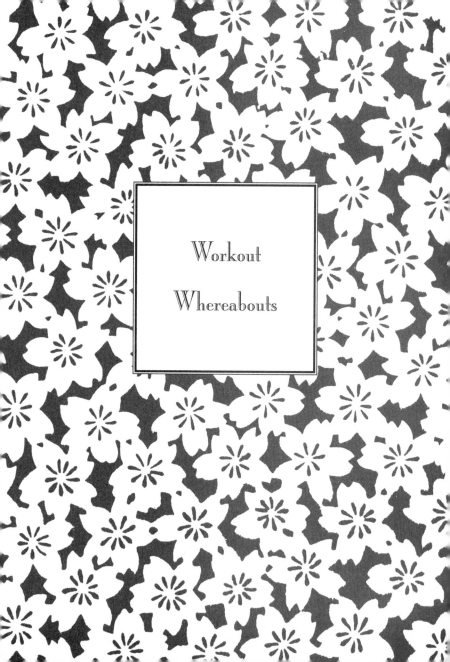

Workout

Whereabouts

# Apex

205 E. 85th St., 2nd Floor  (212) 737-8377
Hours: Monday through Friday 6 AM–9 PM
Saturday and Sunday 8 AM–6 PM

This 10,000-square-foot gym is an inviting place to work out. Bleached wood floors, crisp modern decor, airy exercise and weight rooms, and a never-crowded feel. Things work a bit differently here: there's no yearly membership, and you make appointments for exercise classes the day before. Single visits cost $17 each and a series of 20—which must be used within two months—costs $225. Each visit entitles you to either just use the equipment or take a class and spend 20 minutes using the equipment. Personal trainers are available, as are nutritionists.

After a workout you can sit at tables near the juice bar and do *The New York Times* crossword puzzles—they have a pile of copies— or buy eco-friendly cosmetics and household cleansers at the tiny eco-bazaar.

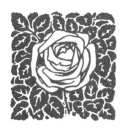

# Back in Shape with Majorie Jaffee

37 W. 54th St. (212) 245-9131

Hours: Monday through Friday 10:30 AM–6:30 PM;
Saturday class at 10:15 AM

Backaches? Pains in the neck? This studio's for you.

Lots of fitness centers offer stretching and strengthening exercises, but this low-key midtown studio specializes in techniques to relieve back and neck pain, improve posture, and increase strength and flexibility. Jaffee was trained by Dr. Sonya Weber, founder of Columbia Presbyterian's Posture and Back Care Clinic, and she served for ten years as head instructor of corrective exercises for the YWCA's Backcare Program. Her classes are small and personal, and attract young and old.

One class per week $16. Each additional class $1 less (two classes per week, $15 each). Private lessons by appointment.

If you're weary of the city and need a break, Jaffee leads groups to Montego Bay, Jamaica, for spa vacations.

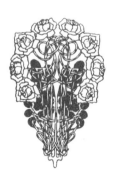

# Body Design by Gilda

187 E. 79th St. (212) 737-8440
Hours: Monday through Friday 6:15 AM–:30 PM;
Saturday and Sunday 8 AM–7 PM

There's no glitz or glamour in this small, two-classroom exercise studio, but from early morning on, seven days a week, the heavy schedule of classes attracts a serious, 30+ crowd of mostly women who are buoyed by the loud music and ready to sweat. There's a large classroom on the second level for 30, and a second, smaller classroom one flight above for 12. The mixed-level classes cover a variety of needs, including step aerobics, body sculpting, muscle beach (a body-sculpting class taught by bodybuilders), active isolated flexibility (a stretch class), and yoga.

The studio also has a small aerobics area (two treadmills, two bikes, two StairMasters) that anyone can use for $10 per half-hour and $15 for one hour.

Classes $15, less when purchased in bulk. (i.e., 30 classes are $300). Newcomers can take a free trial class. Private classes cost $60 in the studio, $75 at home.

# Crunch Fitness

404 Lafayette St., bet. E. 4th and Astor Pl. (212) 614-0120
54 E. 13th St., bet. University Pl. and Broadway (212) 475-2018
162 W. 83rd St., bet. Amsterdam and Columbus Aves. (212) 875-1902
Monday through Friday 6:30 AM–10 PM;
Saturday and Sunday 8 AM–8 PM

The names of the classes—uninhibited funk, brand new butt, hip hop funk, and cuttin' up—tell you most of what you need to know about Crunch. It's a young, hip, fun place to work out. The walls are purple, yellow, red . . . there are banquettes covered in zebra fabric; the lighting is kooky and contemporary; and you can take spinning (exercise-bike work combined with fantasy: you're on a hill, somewhere in France . . .). You can also box, buy fitness clothes, and socialize.

Membership, about $850 a year, but there are often specials starting at about $650. Day passes, $15.

# Equinox Fitness Clubs

344 Amsterdam Ave., bet. 76th and 77th Sts. (212) 721-4200

897 Broadway bet. 19th and 20th Sts. (212) 780-9300

2465 Broadway bet. 91st and 92nd Sts. (212) 799-1818

Hours: Monday through Thursday 5:30 AM–11 PM;

Friday 5:30 AM–10 PM; Saturday and Sunday 8 AM–9 PM

This well-maintained black-and-stainless-steel world of plentiful aerobics equipment, weight machines, free weights, and exercise classes draws a serious as well as social crowd at all hours of the day. The club prides itself on its top fitness instructors (including former club owner Jeff Martin) and its state-of-the-art wellness center which offers chiropractic services, acupuncture, herb therapy, podiatry, hypnosis, and nutrition counseling in addition to facials and massage. The newest club on Broadway, between 91st and 92nd, is scheduled to open on September 15, 1995.

Membership: $295 initiation fee plus monthly dues of $82, or $825 per year. Day passes, $26.

# Gold's Gym

1635 Third Ave. at 91st St. (212) 987-7200
Hours: Monday through Friday 5 AM–midnight;
Saturday and Sunday 6 AM–11 PM

Gold's Gym got its start on the West Coast as a temple for serious bodybuilders. Now there are others worldwide, but this block-long facility on the Upper East Side is Manhattan's first, and the scene is more health club than bodybuilding mecca. On the street level there are two spacious classrooms facing the street, and in the center of the club—unfortunately in an area without windows or view—a large aerobic equipment room, too tightly packed for comfort, with 30 treadmills, 40 exercise bikes, and 35 StairMasters. Downstairs in the basement area are the freeweights, a 50x30 foot swimming pool with six lap lanes, and the locker rooms.

One wonderful amenity is the free baby sitting service for up to two hours, for children ages three months to eight years. This room is bright, clean, and sunny. The club also offers nutrition counseling, fitness evaluations, and massage, the latter at a bargain rate of $40 an hour for members. There are numerous membership options, but basic yearly membership is $889.

# Mary Leck

(212) 666-8125

Hours: By appointment

Leck is a guru of sorts to those in need of mind–body work. She helps tranquilize spirits by teaching yoga breathing, helps increase strength and flexibility with yoga postures and yoga-based exercises, and if tense bodies are still crying out for soothing, she'll rub out tensions with Swedish and shiatsu massage. Leck studied Swedish massage at Esalen and is accredited by the American Oriental Body Therapy Association. Rate: $75 an hour; $80 for home visits plus taxi fare.

# The Lotte Berk Method

23 E. 67th St.  (212) 288-6613
Bridgehampton, spring and summer only  (516) 537-3290
Hours: Monday through Friday 7 AM–7:30 PM;
Saturday 8:30 AM–1 PM; Sunday 9:30 AM–1:15 PM

Think you're in pretty good shape, right? Ha! Take a class at Lotte
Berke, and unless you've been training for triathalons, chances are
you'll feel the burn in your thighs for days to come. In the span of an
hour, the Lotte Berke Method takes you through a program of hatha
yoga stretches, weight work, push-ups, modern dance, ballet barre
work, orthopedic exercises, abdominal crunches, and pelvic thrusts
that tone, stretch, and strengthen muscles. The out-of-shape will feel
like misfits and vow never to go back, but of course they will.

The program was developed by founder Lotte Berk, a German-
Jewish refugee now in her early 80s who lives in London. A former
modern dancer whose performances were banned by the Nazis,  she
escaped with her English husband and later gave up dancing after a
fall.

The system of rehabilitative exercises she designed with an
osteopath became the basis for the program she later taught. Twenty-
five years ago, Lydia Bach bought the rights to Berk's name and
opened the New York studio. Former ballet dancer Elizabeth
Halfpapp and her husband, Fred DeVito, run the studio today. Most
classes are co-ed, and cost $16. There's only a small savings if you
sign up for blocks of 10, 20, or 30 hours.

# Manhattan Body

149 E. 72nd St., 2nd floor  (212) 772-6087

Hours: Monday 8 AM-7:15 PM; Tuesday, Thursday 6:45 AM–7:15 PM;
Wednesday, Friday 8 AM–6:15 PM; Saturday 9 AM–12 PM;
Sunday 9 AM–10:30 AM

Former jazz dancer Ann Piccirillo runs this small, low-key all-women's gym that is popular with locals. There's one classroom, the lighting is kind, and the ages and fitness levels of the regulars are mixed in all classes. You won't find yourself wedged between fitness goddesses in thong leotards who have washboard abs. These are real people—young, old, in- or out-of-shape. There are three types of classes: body toning, step aerobics, and interval step, for the beginning stepper.

The body-toning class is the biggest draw, and the feedback is "there isn't a muscle they miss." This is the class to  contour the body and make you long and lean, says Piccirillo. To ward off boredom, routines are rechoreographed every three months. You can take a free trial class. Individual classes cost $15, but prices go down the more you buy. Two hundred classes cost $1,400, or $7 a class. Private classes in the studio or your home, $60 an hour.

# New York Sports

For information on nearest location (212) 246-6700

Hours: Vary depending on club. Those in residential areas open seven days, Monday through Friday 6 AM–11 PM, Saturday and Sunday 8 AM–9 PM.

New York Sports, owned by Town Sports International, is the largest chain of health clubs in the New York area, with 16 clubs in Manhattan, one in Brooklyn, one in Great Neck, and one in E. Brunswick, N.J. The clubs are clean, modern, comfortably laid out, and offer lots of spanking-new aerobic equipment (including recumbent bikes and Nautilus skate machines), weight machines, and freeweights, as well as classes. Also provided are such amenities as babysitting—$3 an hour—free health lectures, and free body composition testing, offered at various times.

There are several membership options. All include an initiation fee of between $99 and $249 and a monthly fee ranging from $53 to $68.

Membership is "no commitment," which means you don't have to keep paying beyond the first month. But if you do quit and sign up a year later, you have to pay the initiation fee again. The clubs don't offer day passes, but those thinking of joining are generally allowed to try the club for a day at no charge.

# Radu's Physical Culture Studio

24 W. 57th St., 2nd floor  (212) 581-1995
East Hampton  24-26 Gingerbread Lane  (516) 329-0077
Hours: Monday, Wednesday, Friday 7 AM–7 PM; Tuesday and
Thursday 8 AM–7 PM; Saturday and Sunday by appointment

Radu Teodorescu, a former phys-ed teacher and track-and-field coach
in Romania, has established a reputation over the past 20 years as one
of the toughest trainers in town. In his midtown gym you can work
privately with him (or an associate) or take an exhausting hour-long
group class with up to 16 others. Either way, at a peppy pace you'll do
stretching, yoga, jumping, running, weight work, stair-climbing, sit-
ups, and more. (Candice Bergen once said of Radu, "The good news is
it's only an hour.") The other good news is that Radu promises you'll
see results after three weeks if you work out at least three times a
week. Private hour with Radu $100, with one of his associates, $65.
Classes $16. Prices go down the more sessions you buy.

# Reebok Sports Club/NY

160 Columbus Ave. at 67th St.  (212) 362-6800

Hours: Monday through Friday 5:30 AM–11 PM;
Saturday and Sunday 8 AM–8 PM

This limited-membership fitness club one-ups just about every other in town. Operated by the fitness-shoe manufacturer and the creators of the luxe Sports Club/LA, it boasts: a 5,000 square-foot cardiovascular deck with 117 pieces of equipment ◆ a 6-lap to the mile rooftop outdoor running and in-line skating track ◆ a junior Olympic swimming pool ◆ a 45-foot rock-climbing wall ◆ a sports simulation center, including a downhill skiing simulator, a wide-screen golf simulator, windsurfing, and boxing, all with instructional and motivational audio-visual displays ◆ a Kids Only Club with programs for children ages six months to 17 years ◆ nutrition counseling, massage, facials, manicures, and pedicures.

Membership fees subject to change: initiation fee of $950, monthly dues of $135.

# Ravi Singh

THE KUNDALINI YOGA CENTER

401 Lafayette St. at 4th St., 3rd floor  (212) 475-0212

Hours: Afternoon classes:  Monday through Friday at noon;

Evening classes: Monday through Friday at 6 PM;

Tuesday 6:30 PM; weekends: Saturday 11 AM, Sunday 3 PM

And you thought you were breathing well on your own!  Just one session with Singh and you'll be feeling as though you're on an oxygen high. Kundalini yoga is exciting, invigorating, and energizing, combining meditation, static holds, intensive breathing, and aerobic exercises. You walk away with brighter eyes, a clearer head, and an A+ in mental attitude—and that's just from one session in his studio, or via his videotapes, which you can play at home.

One and a quarter-hour class, $10. Sunday classes are two hours and cost $12.

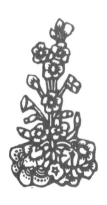

# The Vertical Club

330 E. 61st St., bet. 1st and 2nd Aves. (212) 355-5100
139 W. 32nd St., bet. 6th and 7th Aves. (212) 465-1750
351 W. 49th St., bet. 8th and 9th Aves. (212) 265-9400
335 Madison Ave., on 43rd St. bet. Madison
and Vanderbilt Aves. (212) 983-5320
Hours: All are open seven days, call for individual hours.

This is a health club that has disco/social club in its genes. The main
floor of the flagship 61st St. branch looks like a hotel lobby complete
with tanning salon. Downstairs there's a whirlpool and a three-lane
lap pool. The second floor is dominated by a giant open classroom
and a tightly packed aerobics equipment area, and on a balcony just
above it is the indoor running track outlined in red neon. The five-
level club also boasts indoor and outdoor tennis courts and a clientele
made up of numerous svelte women dressed in racy workout wear.
Diet before you sign up. One-year membership, $1,247; two-year,
$1,599. One-year tennis membership, $3,120. No day passes.

# World Gym

1926 Broadway, bet. 64th and 65th Sts. (212) 874-0942
Hours: Monday through Friday 24 hours;
Saturday and Sunday 7 AM–9 PM

This open, airy gym has a wall of west-facing windows offering a spectacular view of Lincoln Center. The 20,000 square foot, horse-shoe-shaped space houses green and white Cybex machines that invite a workout even if you're not into indoor exercising. There are two rooms offering every imaginable type of class. Just a sampling: boxing, slide board, step, variations on standard aerobics, washboard workout (billed as 30 minutes your stomach won't forget), yoga, Pilates, and even meditation.

And hey—what's bad about working out with the likes of Madonna, Tony Danza, Kathleen Turner, Bruce Springsteen, JFK Jr., and Sharon Stone?

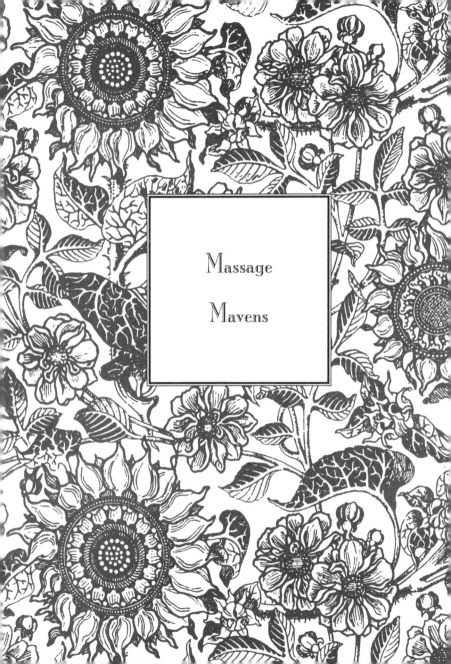

Massage

Mavens

Massage therapists must be licensed and registered by the State Education Department to practice in New York State. To find out if a therapist is licensed, you can call the New York State Education Department, Division of Professional Licensing Services, at (518) 474-3817.

## Tina Awad

W. 15th St. and W. 79th St. studios  (212) 989-5506
Hours: Monday through Saturday 11 AM–7 PM

It's not surprising that Awad, a former dancer, segued into massage feet first. Three weeks after starting a class in reflexology, she took a fall, landed on her tailbone, and found herself in excruciating pain. The next day her reflexology teacher worked on her feet, targeting the treatment to points corresponding to her injured coccyx. Within 24 hours, the pain diminished by 50 percent, Awad said, and she became a convert. After practicing reflexology for two years, Awad went on to get her massage license—that was eight years ago. Since then she has been combining reflexology with body massage and energy-balancing work. She has a varied group of patients ranging from a chef who spends long days on his feet to dancers with injuries, those with pain and scar build-up following foot surgery, and many more with just plain tired feet and bodies.

Rates: $70–$75 per hour, depending on location. One and a half hours $105–$110.

# Patricia Betty

E-SCENTIALLY YOURS, LTD.
THE AROMATHERAPY PLACE
24 E. 38th St., Suite 1A  (212) 545-0229 / 1-800-870-6026
Hours: By appointment, Monday through Saturday 11 AM–9 PM

Every other salon in town boasts of aromatherapy facials and massage, but here is the woman who literally wrote the book. Pat Betty, author, lecturer, and massage therapist for 17 years, now divides her time between giving treatments, teaching aromatherapy, and selling essential oils and perfume oils.

The lush plant life of her native Jamaica sparked Betty's initial interest in herb medicine and biology. Following work as a physical therapist, she began using massage with plant oils for their medicinal benefits.

A treatment begins with a one-hour consultation to determine which oils best suit your needs—she uses five or six oil blends. (She also custom-makes fragrances for clients). A two-hour massage follows, with techniques borrowed from lymphatic drainage work, acupressure, deep-tissue, and Swedish massage. You'll feel so loose and relaxed, you'll slither out the door.

Two-hour aromatherapy massage, $150; one and a quarter-hour aromatherapy facial, $90. Oils available through a mail-order catalog.

# Eastside Massage Therapy Center

351 E. 78th St. (212) 249-2927

Hours: Monday through Friday 11 AM–9:30 PM; Saturday 9 AM–7 PM

"People who come here are not looking for a spa experience," says Robin Ehrlich Bragdon, the massage therapist who heads this Upper East Side studio with her husband, Stuart. The approach here is clinical, and each of the eight therapist starts with your medical history. Massage concentrates on specific problem areas. The majority of clients come in with back and neck problems, tight shoulders, muscle spasms, or pinched nerves, says Bragdon, who calls the neck, shoulders, and lower back "the New York stress points."

Among the offerings: Swedish, therapeutic, and medical massage (for specific conditions such as sciatica or shin splints), deep-muscle therapy, and lymphatic drainage to reduce inflammation and fluid build-up. Stuart Bragdon specializes in massage therapy for sports and dance injuries.

One unusual therapy by Bragdon—who lectures on medical massage at Sloan Kettering Cancer Center—is the very delicate Dr. Vodder method of manual lymph drainage massage, used after plastic surgery. She says it enhances healing by helping fluids to drain, scars to heal more quickly, and bruises to disappear faster.

One-hour massage, $60. Ten massages, $540. Massage with Bragdon, $95. House calls without table, $85. House calls with table, $100 plus taxi fare.

# Charles Haack

(212) 673-8324

Hours: By appointment

Haack is a dancer as well as a massage therapist, so he knows first-hand the effects of overexertion, pains, sprains, fatigue, and both physical and psychological stress. He has toured as massage therapist with the Joffrey Ballet and with Mikhail Baryshnikov's White Oak Dance Project, and after you've had just one treatment it's easy to see why he would be favored by dancers. Haack uses mostly Swedish techniques, and he works deeply and strongly on muscles, using long, continuous stretching, elongating movements. He doesn't miss a muscle—from head to toes—and at the end of the session when he says, "Take your time getting up," you'll wonder whether your legs can support you.

One-hour massage in his East Village studio, $50. One and a half hours, $75. House calls without table, $90. House calls with table, $85 plus cab fare. House calls for two people: second massage costs $50.

# Greer Jonas

(212) 769-2345

Hours: By appointment, Tuesday through Saturday 8 AM–6 PM

An aromatherapy massage with Jonas—who works from her Upper West Side studio—is often an eclectic blend of techniques, including Swedish, deep-muscle, polarity, reflexology, myofascial release, and craniosacral, the latter a nouveau type of therapy involving various methods of cradling the head and sacral area, at the bottom of the spine.

Is the pressure comfortable? She wants your feedback. "I'm always telling the client, "You know more than I do." If there's pain you're going to restrict yourself, so it's important that the client communicates."

Since the oils she'll use depend on what you say, tell her if your chest and sinuses are congested, if your muscles ache, or if your spirits need lifting. She'll use eucalyptus or lavender, for example, because they're decongestants, rosemary on your legs because, she says, it works on toxins and cellulite, and if it's summer, maybe some lemon and grapefruit oil because of their euphoric effects.

One-hour massage, $65; one and a half hours, $85. Men by referral only.

# Ken Kobayashi

143 E. 35th St. (212) 685-4325

Hours: By appointment, Monday through Friday 10 AM-6 PM

Don't be put off by the less-than-pristine appearance of this Murray Hill townhouse. Yes, it looks musty and East Village. And in case you were wondering, the strange collection of gnarled roots sitting in the glass bottles along the walls are desiccated herbs. Translation: herbal remedies.

Unless plush surroundings are the *sine qua non* of a massage experience for you, stay put. Kobayashi, a Japanese shiatsu expert and healer who claims to have worked on over a million people, knows his way around your meridians. Trained from boyhood by his family, he swears he can sense disease, improve back pain, and banish a host of evils. He'll pull, press, elbow, and massage you—and admittedly there are uncomfortable moments—but 75 minutes later, you'll float out like a cloud. Stress? What's that?

Kobayashi also teaches breathing classes based on an old Chinese technique. After only a few weeks you'll look ten years younger, he says. Yes! Shiatsu massage, $90. (Unlike other shiatsu practitioners cited in this section, Kobayashi is not licensed in New York, although he says he holds Japanese licenses for acupuncture and massage. I feel his expertise warrants inclusion.)

## Leslie Leonelli

155 W. 71st St. (212) 769-1511

Hours: By appointment, Monday through Saturday 10:30 AM-8 PM

Leonelli treats all-over tension with a soothing Swedish body massage, works on problem areas with medical massage, does polarity therapy for energy balancing, and will treat just about any condition for which massage is appropriate. But she's also built up a reputation among the cognoscenti in the arts world for her massage therapy for singers. This treatment works the neck, head, and face, the front and back of the torso, and the spine, and is designed to increase vocal clarity and resonance by releasing tightness in the upper body, specifically the throat, the tongue, the sinuses, and the chest area.

One-hour massage, $60; half-hour massage, $35.

## Laura Norman and Associates

41 Park Ave., bet. 36th and 37th Sts. (212) 532-4404

Sag Harbor (516) 725-4440

Hours: By appointment

Laura Norman is a licensed massage therapist, who's studied Shiatsu and other bodywork disciplines, but after practicing reflexology for almost 25 years, she's convinced that it gives better results than any other type of body work. Norman's technique borrows from several disciplines: Swedish, shiatsu, Traeger, stretching, polarity, aromatherapy, and homeopathy.

Over the course of a session she massages fragrant lotions into the feet and works the 7,000+ nerve endings in each foot that correspond to every body part, lulling you into a dreamlike state. If you happen to have a foot injury and can't have your feet done, Norman will apply the same therapy to your hands.

Reflexology can help a host of ailments rooted in stress and tension, Norman maintains, such as PMS, aches and pains, digestive problems, sinus woes, and headaches. Norman also offers courses in reflexology leading to certification—not the equivalent of New York State licensing, however.

A 45-minute session with Norman, $100; 30 minutes, $65. A 45-minute session with an associate, $75; 30 minutes with an associate, $55.

## Kathy Rabbers

(718) 596-3070

Hours: Monday in her Greenwich Village studio 10 AM–7 PM; Tuesday through Friday, house calls only; and Sunday in her studio 10 AM–8 PM

Kathy Rabbers isn't the therapist to visit if you have an injury or need a specific type of medical massage. But if you have tight shoulders and an aching neck, or suffer from stress overload, she's just a phone call away.

After 15 years in practice, Rabbers has developed a unique massage style, combining Swedish, pressure-point, and craniosacral therapy. The hour goes by in a flash; there's a lot of stationary pressure, head-holding, body-cradling, not a lot of rubbing, stroking, or tapping. Still, sixty minutes later, you're calm. How did she do that?

Hour massage, $65. House calls, $100.

# The Stress Less Step

48 E. 61st St. (212) 826-6222

Hours: Monday through Friday 9 AM-11 PM. First appointment at 10, last appointment 9:30; Saturday and Sunday 8:30 AM–10 PM. First appointment at 9:30, last appointment 8:30.

Just get past the sage and cedar incense cloud—"clearing negative energy"—that can fell you when you open the door to this massage studio early in the morning. And pay no mind to the New Age books and tapes for sale, such as "You Are the Ocean." You're not the ocean. You don't make waves. And this is not Haight-Ashbury circa 1970. You're just a world-weary soul in need of healing hands, yes? You're in the right place.

This midtown salon, across the street from the power-breakfast Regency Hotel, offers a team of talented therapists with an extensive range of specialties, starting with the usual—Swedish, Shiatsu, and Russian sports massage—to strange, stranger, and strangest modalities, such as polarity, Reiki, and MariEl (all somewhat mystifying regimens—à la holding the hands above the body —designed to balance energy). The spa also offers facials and bodywraps, hypnosis, and creative visualization.

Hour massage, $60. No tipping permitted.

# Swedish Institute

226 W. 26th St., bet. 7th and 8th Aves. (212) 924-0991
Hours: Monday 9 AM–12 PM and 1:15 PM–4:15 PM;
Wednesday 9 AM–12 PM and 6 PM–9 PM

Those with letters of referral from MDs or chiropractors prescribing massage for conditions such as sciatica or lower-back pain can get bargain-priced massages by third-semester students. Those who pass muster sign up for eight consecutive weeks of massage and come once or twice a week for either half-hour or hour massages with the same therapist. (Students then do a research paper on the client's ailment.) The clinic accommodates up to 27 people, and massages are given in three large rooms with individual tables sectioned off with curtains.

A series of eight half-hour massages, $95; eight one-hour massages, $190.

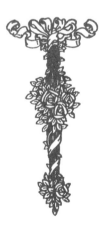

# Joan Witkowski

(212) 620-0308

Hours: By appointment only, Tuesday through Saturday 10 AM-8 PM

Witkowski has a large following of regular clients who come to her West Village studio for deep-muscle therapy. They come with injuries, with tight backs and necks, with frozen shoulders, painful knees, tension headaches, sciatica, and a host of other ills that respond to her stroking, pulling, pushing, and prodding. Working with the aid of an infrared lamp, she lubricates the skin with essential oils, presses to the limits of comfort—but not beyond—and eases tight and troubled tendons, ligaments, and muscles that may have been injured or are just painfully strained and misaligned due to bad posture, bad habits, and bad karma. When problems have eased, her regulars keep coming to enjoy the benefits of preventive stroking. A 55-minute session, $85.

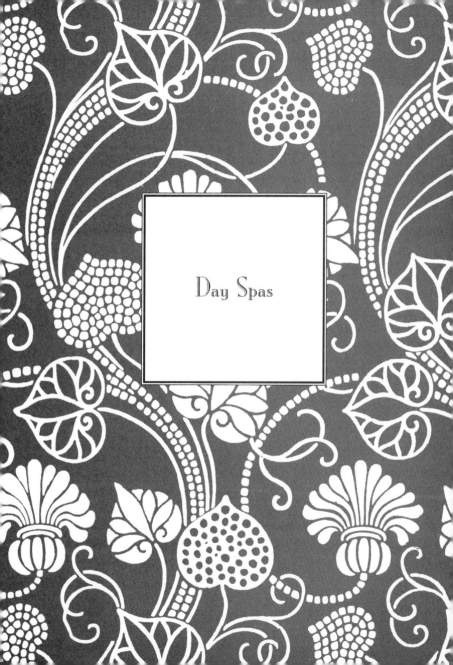

# Day Spas

# Elizabeth Arden

THE SALON

691 Fifth Ave., bet. 54th and 55th Sts. (212) 546-0200

Hours: Monday, Tuesday, and Friday 8 AM–6 PM; Wednesday 8 AM–7:30 PM; Thursday 8 AM–8 PM; Sunday 9 AM–4 PM

This grande dame of day spas, opened in 1929, still graciously offers an oasis of calm amid the bustle of New York life and provides a wide variety of services, including face treatments (from the mundane deep cleansing to exotic enzyme peels, and the CACI treatment, which some dub "passive exercise" or "nonsurgical face lift"); apothecary face treatments using herbs, minerals, vitamins, and aromatic oils; massage; herbal bodywraps; waxing; haircutting; hair coloring; scalp treatments; manicures; pedicures; and makeup.

While prices are moderate ($50 for an hour of massage, $60 for a deep-cleansing facial), the best buys are the packages, such as the Arden Beauty Basics which includes a facial, manicure, and pedicure for $85, and the series of services, such as ten massages for $450.

To accommodate busy schedules, services begin by appointment at 7 AM . Local phone and fax services are free.

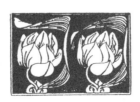

# Dorit Baxter

SKIN CARE, BEAUTY AND DAY SPA
47 W. 57th St. (212) 371-4542
Hours: Monday through Saturday 9 AM–9 PM

Full salon services are available at this midtown spa in addition to some unique face and body treatments. The Solar Energy Mud Treatment, for example, is an hour and a half of indulgence, beginning with one half-hour of massage, the application of mud from the Dead Sea, a facial massage, a facial mask, and then a warm shower ($90). This one treatment, boasts Israeli owner Dorit Baxter, "relaxes, exfoliates the skin, increases circulation, draws out impurities, and relaxes muscles." Regulars swear by it.

Another Baxter special is the Dead Sea Salt Body Scrub, $40. For half an hour, a paste of sea salt and aromatic oils (rosemary, lavender, and mint) is massaged into the skin. A soapless shower follows, and *voilà*, the skin is silky-smooth. Baxter says she uses this rejuvenating rub to counter the effects of jet lag. (Just one caution: Don't shave your legs the morning of the treatment or the salt will sting.)

Still another special is the "organic waxing," done with a gentle product that doesn't cause the typical kinds of adverse reactions (irritation, rashes, ingrown hairs) that can be produced by other waxes, Baxter says. It's particularly suited to the face, underarm, and bikini areas. Prices start at $10.

# Georgette Klinger

978 Madison Avenue, between 76th and 77th Sts. (212) 744-6900

501 Madison Ave., bet. 52nd and 53rd Sts. (212) 838-3200

1-800-KLINGER

Hours: Monday, Wednesday, Friday 9 AM–6 PM; Tuesday, Thursday 9 AM–8:30 PM; Saturday 8:30 AM–5:30 PM; Sunday 9 AM–6 PM (only 501 Madison is open)

Czech-born Georgette Klinger opened her first skin care salon in New York in 1940, and over a half-century later business is booming, catering to 200 clients a day. Facials are the most popular treatment—Hilary Clinton has been going to esthetician Maria Colda for more than a decade—but the body treatments are the perfect Rx for those who yearn to relax and be coddled.

The one-hour Revitalizing Body Treatment ($75), for example, begins with an exfoliating massage using an oatmeal–almond peeling cream. Next, cocoa butter is applied to the dry areas, the entire body is wrapped in warm towels soaked in an herbal extract (chamomile, eucalyptus, lavender) and then covered with plastic, a sheet, and a heated blanket. After you spend 20 minutes in soothing darkness, the wrappings are removed and your body is sprayed with rosewater and massaged with an herbal lotion. You emerge almost giddy and are offered a generous mug of herbal tea served with wheat biscuits. (Book with Tina—she's wonderful.)

Other services: massage, hair care, manicures, pedicures, and waxing. The uptown salon has a men's skin-care clinic.

TO SAVE MONEY: Buy services in packages, or wait for the sales in December and especially August.

# Millefleurs

6 Varick St., corner of Franklin St.   (212) 966-3656
Hours: Seven days, 9 AM–11 PM


This downtown day spa (recently moved to the above address), has a holistic bent that appeals to the lower Manhattan audience it caters to. It has a global perspective of health and beauty, according to owner and licensed acupuncturist Gina Michael, and offers facials, massage, reflexology, acupuncture, herbal wraps—perhaps the best known of its treatments, done with a solution made with 111 herbs, minerals, and seaweed ($75)—sea-salt scrubs, sage foot wraps, hair services, manicures, pedicures, and for the cleanliness-obsessed, even colonics.

The new 2,500-square-foot space patterns itself after an ancient Egyptian temple, with waterfalls, reflecting pools, thrones, and the like. The only thing you won't do is cruise home along the Nile.


# Peninsula Spa

700 Fifth Ave. at 55th St., 21st floor   (212) 903-3910
Hours: Monday through Friday 6 AM–10 PM; Saturday, Sunday
8:30 AM–7:30 PM  (treatments start at 8:45 AM on all days)


Exit on the 21st floor of this opulent midtown hotel and you're at the reception desk of one of Manhattan's poshest spas. Operated independently of the hotel by Club Sports International, this luxe facility decorated in beige, green, and dark polished wood is a tranquil oasis high above the madding crowds below.

Services include an exotic menu of facials, aromatherapy treatments, massage, manicures, and pedicures. Go up the interior staircase for classes, aerobics equipment, (alas, this room should be twice the size), workouts with personal trainers, nutrition counseling, hair services in the separate Melange Salon, outdoor sunning on decks with river-to-river views, and swimming in a pool surrounded by sublime city vistas. Membership prices? Sky-high to match.

But you don't have to belong to the club to come just for a treatment—and these range from about $75 to $90. Get three treatments and you're entitled to use the pool and equipment, and take classes. Regulars don't bother to bring their own workout clothes—the club provides t-shirts, shorts, and socks. Hate to carry your running shoes? A fee of $15 a month buys them a Fifth Ave. address.

Membership in this triplex fitness aerie: Individual: $2,600 initiation fee plus $180 monthly dues. Husband and wife, $2,900 initiation fee plus $260 monthly dues.

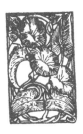

Department Store

Beauty

# Barneys

660 Madison Ave. at 61 st St.  (212) 826-8900
Hours: Monday through Friday 10 AM–8 PM; Saturday 10 AM–7 PM;
Sunday 12 PM-6 PM
106 Seventh Ave. at 17th St.  (212) 929-9000
Hours: Monday through Thursday 10 AM–9 PM;
Friday 10 AM–8 PM; Saturday 10 AM–7 PM; Sunday 12 PM–6 PM
2 World Financial Center, mezzanine level
(LOOK cosmetics only)  (212) 945-1600
Hours: Monday through Friday 10 AM–7 PM;
Saturday 10 AM–6 PM; Sunday 12 PM–5 PM

Barneys has some unique offerings in its cosmetics department in the
back of the mosaic-tiled main floor of the Madison Ave. store. Pull
up your collar to keep out the snooty chill in the air, then stroll the
aisles and you'll come upon makeup by Poppy (from Australia); Shu
Uemura; Molton Brown; Stila; Nars, by makeup artist François
Nars; Make Up For Ever; Face Stockholm (the only other place
this line is sold in New York is at Face Stockholm—see p. 18—but
Barneys prices are higher); and Barneys own pricy LOOK line.

Head to the back of the cosmetics area and you'll find Route du
Thè, the store's own fragrance, redolent of green apples and lily of
the valley, 3.4 ozs. for $48; Valobra soaps; Coudray body cream;
LeClerc powders; and some neat gift items, such as makeup brushes
with fat handles made from multicolored femo clay resembling the
patterns of Venetian glass beads.

Barneys offers free messenger service in Manhattan for orders of $50 or more, purchased with a Barneys charge card. Without the Barneys card there is a $7 charge.

Coming soon: an in-store gymnasium and spa to open on the 8th Floor of the Madison Ave. store, along with another Roger Thompson hair salon, so uptown Thompson clients won't have to journey down to 17th St. for haircuts.


## Bergdorf Goodman (see also p. 35 and p. 46)

1 W. 57th St. (212) 753-7300
Hours: Monday through Saturday 10 AM–6 PM;
Thursday 10 AM–8 PM


There is an inviting opulence to this store, and the main floor cosmetics department is no exception. Most of the traditional prestige lines are here, as well as Laszlo, Sisley, Guerlain, Kiehl, Origins, the popular Bobbi Brown, and Philip B., a botanical line of hair and body products. Purchases can be messengered to Manhattan addresses for $12.50.

Head up to the seventh floor to the Frederic Fekkai Beauty Center (Martha Stewart does) for beauty services. While most of the operators here are top-notch, salon prices tend to be high, and the tempo can be frenetic. If your idea of a good time is watching who comes in, and enjoying the sight of Ms. You-Know-Who walk in with her pet cocker spaniel, you'll have a fine old time while your nails dry ($21-$26 for manicures, $45 for pedicures).

Haircut with Fekkai $290; with "hair designers" $150; with senior stylists $110; with junior stylists $90. Single-process color $65 and up; highlights with junior stylists $135 and up; with senior stylists $200. Other services: facials $90; massage $90; makeup; waxing.

# Bloomingdale's

1000 Third Ave., bet. 59th and 60th Sts.
Customer Service (212) 355-5900
Hours: Monday through Friday 10 AM–8:30 PM;
Saturday 10 AM–7 PM; Sunday 11 AM–7 PM

This home away from home for New York women has an impressive collection of prestigious lines of cosmetics—Yves St. Laurent, Christian Dior, Lauder, Lancôme, Lancaster, La Prairie, Origins, Janet Sartin, and Fashion Fair, to name just a few—and a newcomer to the market called Studio Gear, a professional line that echos M.A.C. cosmetics that was started just over a year ago by Steve Rohr, who worked for M.A.C.'s distributor, International Prestige Products.

Near and yet a world apart from the buzzing activity of the main floor is a bountiful offering of minispas: The Chanel Treatment Room; The Estée Lauder Spa; the Christian Dior Centre de Beauté; Lancôme's Institut de Beauté; and Adrien Arpel.

The Chanel Treatment Room is tucked away on the balcony just above the Chanel cosmetics area and offers plush surroundings with soundproof rooms. Services include a number of hour-and-a-quarter facials for $70 or $80; a 45-minute minifacial for $45; a one-hour makeup lesson for $37.50; and body waxing.

At The Estée Lauder Spa you can choose from a nice package of offerings, ranging from facials, body treatments, massage, manicures, pedicures, makeup, and waxing to combination treatments  such as the two-and-a-half-hour Spa Express, which includes a facial, a massage, and a makeup for $90; and the five-and-a-half-hour day of beauty, which includes a facial, body massage, manicure, pedicure, hand and foot treatment, makeup, and a light lunch, $175.

At the Christian Dior Centre de Beauté, on the balcony just above the Dior costume jewelry department, the menu includes face and body treatments (facials are $70 for women, $55 for men, and $55 for younger skin), makeup lessons, and waxing.

Lancôme's Institut de Beauté, two levels below the main floor, offers a 90-minute "problem solver" facial for extremely dry or very oily skin for $68; a one-hour basic facial with makeup application for $75; makeovers; "colour design;" makeup application; and honey waxing.

The treatment area behind the Adrien Arpel counter offers hour-long facials for $45; deep-cleansing half hours for $25; makeup applications for $25; hour makeup lessons redeemable in products for $50; and waxing. All spas have the same hours as the store.

Want phone help? Bloomingdale's Beauty at Your Service (212-705-2333) will give you beauty assistance in the store or over the phone. They'll also make appointments for beauty services in the store—or outside for services not offered in Bloomingdale's—and send cosmetics by UPS, or messenger them to Manhattan addresses. Messenger service costs $15 weekdays, $20 on weekends.

# Henri Bendel

712 Fifth Ave, bet. 55th and 56th Sts. (212) 247-1100
Hours: Monday, Tuesday, Wednesday, Friday, and Saturday
10 AM–7 PM; Thursday 10 AM–8 PM; Sunday 12 PM–6 PM

Henri Bendel has always been a specialized small-scale department store combining a stylish collection of boutiques. The cosmetics department is on the main floor, and it is limited to just a few choice names such as Chanel, Trish McEvoy, M.A.C., and the new line on the block, LORAC—the oil-free skin treatment line with color cosmetics that California makeup artist Carol Shaw started with "matte and moist lipsticks named for the stars who really use them— "Geena" (Davis), "Demi" (Moore), "Farrah" (Fawcett), and "Angelica" (Houston). The lipsticks sell for $18.50.

If you're in the market for a fragrance that none of your friends will be able to instantly identify, Bendel carries several small, appealing boutique lines such as Annick Goutal, L'artisan Parfum, Maitre Parfum et Gantier, Terra Nova, and Erbe.

Small and exclusive are fitting terms for the third floor Garren salon. A favorite of the editorial crowd, Garren charges a hair-raising $300 for a haircut. Cuts with his associates range from $100 to $200. The salon does coloring; straightening; manicures, $25; pedicures, $40; and polish change, $15 and up.

# Lord & Taylor

424 Fifth Ave., bet. 38th and 39th Sts. (212) 391-3344

Hours: Monday and Tuesday 10 AM–7 PM; Wednesday through
Friday 10 AM–8:30 PM; Saturday 9 AM–7 PM; Sunday 11 AM–6 PM

No exotic lines of cosmetics here—think of it as a comfortable, more
middle-America type of department store—but you can pick up all
the staples: Lauder, Borghese, Chanel, and the like, and the lighting
is so good you don't have to walk outside to get a reading on the color
of your lipstick. The beauty salon, recently taken over by Elizabeth
Arden, is in the back of the main floor up a flight of stairs, and it
offers a wide range of services at downright reasonable prices. A
haircut is $45, a manicure $12, and a pedicure $25. A deep cleansing
facial costs $50, a men's facial $45, and a makeup lesson $50. The
salon also does waxing.

## Macy's Herald Square

151 W. 34th St.

Switchboard: (212) 695-4400

The Beauty Spa: (212) 494-2170

Hours: Monday, Thursday, and Friday 10 AM-8:30 PM;

Tuesday, Wednesday and Saturday 10 AM-7 PM; Sunday 11 AM-7 PM.


The main floor of the world's largest department store is a long walk around if you're trying to compare one company's selection of pink lipsticks to another's. In addition to cosmetics, the main floor is home to Adrien Arpel and the Lancôme Institut de Beauté, where you can have facials, a makeup, or waxing.

For more extensive services in a more traditional salon setting, head up to the fourth floor to The Beauty Spa. Prices are moderate, and the salon offerings range from a haircut ($35) and a manicure ($12) to a corrective facial ($50), a problem skin treatment ($38), and microtreatments, such as Eye Area Rescue—"smoothes, soothes and relaxes eyes" ($12); or the "V" Area Rescue to smooth and remoisturize the throat and under the chin, and the upper chest ($12). The salon also offers makeup application, lessons, and waxing.

Macy's has a small wig department in the back of the seventh floor on the Broadway side, but it's very limited in scope. There are five styles of inexpensive human-hair wigs ranging in price from $60 to $150 and synthetic wigs ranging from $200 to $500.

# Saks Fifth Avenue (see also p. 41)

611 Fifth Ave., bet. 49th and 50th Sts. (212) 753-4000
Hours: Monday, Tuesday, Wednesday, Friday and Saturday
10 AM–6:30 PM; Thursday 10 AM–8 PM; Sunday 12 PM–6 PM
Roppatte's hours: Monday through Friday 6:30 AM–9 PM

The main floor cosmetics department of Saks offers a cornucopia of fine lines of cosmetics, including Yves St. Laurent, Sisley, Nina Ricci, Bobbi Brown, Orlane, La Prairie, Erno Laszlo, M.A.C., and Penhaligon's, the upper-crust British line of scents, cosmetics, shaving apparatus, and accessories for men and women.

If you want to take a sybaritic hour out of a shopping day, head up to the small Institute di Saturnia Spa on the fifth floor for massage, $35–$70; body treatments, $75–$80; facials, $45–$85; and waxing. For hair and skin care, manicures and pedicures, head to the ninth floor. The Salon is a larger, more luxurious beauty emporium presided over by style director Vincent Roppatte. Roppatte's regulars swear by his cutting and coloring expertise, and once a client always a client. Feel free to ask Roppatte about your makeup and your clothes as well as your hair—he's a great resource.

Haircuts: with Roppatte, $125; other stylists, $70. Haircoloring: single process, $65 and up. Highlights: With Roppatte, $250–$300; with other stylists, $150 and up. Manicure, $15; pedicure, $32. Other services: facials, waxing, electrolysis.

Want to get beauty help by phone? Saks' One on One shopping service has a makeup artist on staff. You can reach Christine York at (212) 940-4145 for advice, and then have cosmetics mailed to you, or for $10.95 they can be sent by messenger to your Manhattan address.

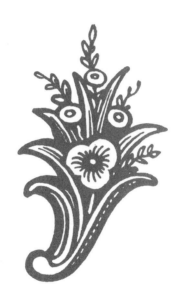

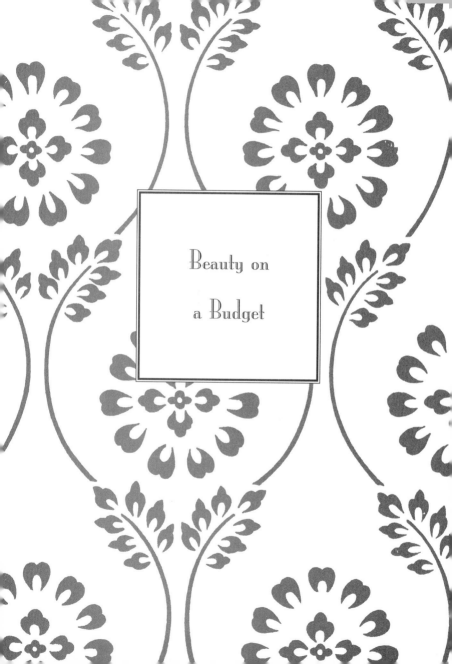

Beauty on

a Budget

Tally up the cost of buying beauty products, going for regular facials, haircuts, haircoloring, manicures, pedicures, exercise, and massage, and one's beauty budget can reach extravagant proportions. Still, there are ways to skimp and save without paying a price in terms of your looks. Following are tips for stretching your beauty dollars:

## Buying cosmetics and fragrances:

You don't have to spend a fortune on makeup to get top-quality products. Buy from mass-market giants such as L'Oreal, Coty, Maybelline, Max Factor, and Revlon, for example, and you'll get quality at low cost. If you do decide to splurge on, say, a foundation from a prestigious line, first see if samples are available at the counter before you plunk down $35 or more for an ounce. If the product doesn't live up to your expectations, return it, and tell the company why.

Check out the discount stores (see Beauty Supplies and Fragrances) before you buy at department stores. Many of the top lines can be found at discount outlets at savings of up to 50 percent.

Never buy fragrances at list price unless you've called around to discounters and found that the scent you're looking for isn't available.

Don't throw out the remains of lipsticks and blushers. Do what models and makeup artists do: scoop out the leftovers and place them in small compartmentalized boxes.

Take advantage of the expertise of makeup artists at the cosmetics counters of department stores. No purchases are required and you can get great advice on your best colors and the types of formulations that will work for you.

## Hair care:

Training nights at hair salons can offer terrific services at rock bottom prices. Frequent the ones where the superstar owners oversee the sessions.

If you're fearful of being a training-night guinea pig, just show up and watch. It will soon become clear who are the most skilled trainees.

If you're not happy with a haircut or haircoloring, speak up. Most salons will fix the job at no charge to you.

Many haircutters invite clients to come into the salon between haircuts to have their bangs trimmed free of charge. This can lengthen the time between haircuts by at least two weeks.

When you're having your hair done at a salon, don't be shy about asking what things cost. During a hair wash, operators may ask if you want your hair conditioned, but fail to inform you if there's an extra charge. It's dismaying for those on a budget to later find that the conditioning treatment added $10 dollars to the cost of the haircut.

Even if you can't afford to book a haircoloring appointment with a superstar operator, you may still be able to book a consultation for no charge or for a fee that can be applied to a service performed by a junior operator.

If your haircoloring budget is slim, opt for treatments such as highlighting rather than single-process color. You can stretch the amount of time between highlighting sessions from two to four months, whereas with single-process color the need for touch ups is obvious in just a few weeks.

Once your hair is colored, lengthen the time between visits by using appropriate shampoos and sun protection products to maintain the vibrancy of the color.

## Skin care:

Regular facials can be expensive. Some skin care salons offer supervised treatments with students at bargain prices.

Ask your esthetician about a discount on your facial if you bring a friend for a treatment.

If your skin does require regular facials, see if you can get a discount by committing to a certain number of treatments.

# Nails:

While weekly manicures are a nice indulgence, you really don't need to go that often. You can stretch the amount of time between manicures by a week or two by opting for pale-colored polish or by buffing your nails lightly. Once your nails are properly shaped, you can maintain the shape with careful filing.

Talk to your manicurist about a discount on manicures if you opt not to have your nails polished, thereby shortening the time the manicure will take.

Beware of extra manicure costs that operators commonly don't tell you about up front. Some salons, for example, tack on a few dollars if you soak your nails in cream rather than water, or if you use Nailtique as a topcoat instead of a cheaper brand.

# Exercise:

Health club membership is a wonderful indulgence, but clearly you can stay fit without signing up. Schedule regular walks or runs in your neighborhood, and buy some light weights to increase the intensity of simple toning exercises that you can do at home.

The yearly cost of health club membership may be beyond your budget, but a far cheaper option is a monthly membership or quarter-year membership just to get you through the coldest winter months.

At the very least, you can buy individual day passes at many clubs for about $15—perfect for inclement weather.

Even if you can't afford costly exercise equipment, you may be able to afford to rent a stationary bike or treadmill for the worst winter months, when snow and ice make it difficult to exercise outdoors.

Before signing up for exercise classes, make sure to ask if you can take a free class first to see if you're comfortable with the routines and the amount of attention you get from the instructor.

## Massage:

Massage schools offer deeply discounted treatments with students if you have any type of medical condition that would benefit from massage.

Massage is costly, but you can save 10–20 percent at some salons by buying a series of treatments.

Massages at home are the ultimate indulgence, but to reduce the price try to get a friend who lives nearby to book a massage the same evening. Some therapists offer reduced rates if their trip to your area means two hours of work rather than one.

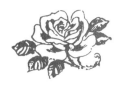

## About the Author

Deborah Blumenthal has been on the beauty beat for fifteen years and was a beauty and fitness columnist for *The New York Times Magazine*. A registered nutritionist, she has written extensively on beauty, fitness, health, and consumer issues for many national newspapers and magazines.

Deborah's first children's book, *The Chocolate Covered Cookie Tantrum*, will be published by Clarion in 1996. She lives in New York with her husband and two daughters.